Reforming
America's
Health Care System

The Hoover Institution gratefully acknowledges
the following individuals and foundations
for their significant support of the
Working Group on Health Care Policy
and this publication:

JAN AND JIM BOCHNOWSKI
LYNDE AND HARRY BRADLEY FOUNDATION

Reforming
America's
Health Care System

The Flawed Vision of ObamaCare

Edited by
Scott W. Atlas, MD

CONTRIBUTING AUTHORS

Scott W. Atlas, MD
Richard A. Epstein
Nadeem Esmail
Helen Evans
Scott Gottlieb, MD
Douglas Holtz-Eakin
Roger Stark, MD
Grace-Marie Turner
Glen Whitman

HOOVER INSTITUTION PRESS
STANFORD UNIVERSITY   STANFORD, CALIFORNIA

The Hoover Institution on War, Revolution and Peace, founded
at Stanford University in 1919 by Herbert Hoover, who went on
to become the thirty-first president of the United States, is an
interdisciplinary research center for advanced study on domestic
and international affairs. The views expressed in its publications are
entirely those of the authors and do not necessarily reflect the views
of the staff, officers, or Board of Overseers of the Hoover Institution.

www.hoover.org

Hoover Institution Press Publication No. 602
Hoover Institution at Leland Stanford Junior University,
Stanford, California, 94305-6010

First printing 2010
16   15   14   13   12   11   10   7   6   5   4   3   2   1

Manufactured in the United States of America

The paper used in this publication meets the minimum
Requirements of the American National Standard for
Information Sciences—Permanence of Paper for Printed
Library Materials, ANSI/NISO Z39.48-1992. ♾

Cataloging-in-Publication Data is available from Library of Congress
ISBN-13: 978-0-8179-1274-1 (cloth.: alk. paper)
ISBN-13: 978-0-8179-1276-5 (e-book)

*To my children, Joe and Ben, who,
I hope, will remain free from governmental intrusion
to be able to exercise personal choices
in pursuit of good health.*

CONTENTS

FOREWORD

THE DEBATE over the direction of U.S. health care policy continues to occupy center stage in the domestic policy arena and will be prominent in the policy debate for many years to come. In March 2010 Congress passed President Obama's legislation to fundamentally transform America's health care platform in the Patient Protection and Affordable Care Act (PPACA). The plan, also referred to as ObamaCare, radically changes health care availability and delivery in the United States, thus affecting the composition and structure of health insurance benefits for individuals, families, and businesses. The promise of future medical advances stemming from the mapping of the human genome, nanotechnology, and other innovations is bright. But progress will require us to transcend the terms of the current debate, which are often expressed as the competing goals of universal insurance and cost control. The aim of the Hoover Institution's Working Group on Health Care Reform is to devise public policies that enable more Americans to get better value for their health care dollar and foster appropriate innovations that extend and improve life. Key principles guiding the group's policy formation include focusing on the central role of individual choice and competitive markets in financing and delivering health services, individual responsibility for health behaviors and decision-making and appropriate guidelines for government intervention in health care markets. The current core membership of this working group includes Scott W. Atlas, John F. Cogan, R. Glenn Hubbard, Daniel P. Kessler, Mark V. Pauly, and Charles E. Phelps.

In this volume, *Reforming America's Health Care System*, Scott Atlas and other health policy experts from the United States, Canada, and Western Europe discuss an array of expectations and alternatives to the health reform legislation that should be considered. Because many important aspects of the legislation do not go into effect until 2014, there is ample time to contribute to the ongoing health care debate.

John Raisian
Tad and Diane Taube Director,
Hoover Institution, Stanford University
Stanford, California

PREFACE

A HIGHLY PARTISAN Democrat-dominated Congress passed President Barack Obama's sweeping legislation to fundamentally transform America's health care in the Patient Protection and Affordable Care Act (PPACA) in March of 2010. The plan the president sought, known as ObamaCare, radically changes health care in the United States, audaciously imposing a strong-armed federal government onto perhaps the most personal of all segments of American life. Americans will be forced to buy insurance they may not want or value; businesses will be fined unless they acquiesce to government dictates about the composition, structure, and breadth of health insurance benefits; coverage must be certified as acceptable by government, not by the individuals and their families who receive the insurance; private insurance companies will be forced to price their products according to government fiat, rather than market forces; and doctors will be compelled to accept lower prices for medical care based solely on what bureaucrats determine to be appropriate.

In addition to the dramatic shift of power from individuals to the federal government, the plan significantly expands eligibility for government insurance like Medicaid. This irrational expansion of an entitlement health insurance program—one that is already failing and widely acknowledged as financially unsustainable—will also conjure up massive tax increases, including taxes on insurance itself as well as on the very sources of innovative medical technology that have improved and prolonged the lives of Americans so dramatically since the previous era.

Inexplicably, the facts published in the world's top medical journals about our system continue to be ignored:

- Americans have the best survival rates from cancer and most serious diseases, and the most rapid decline in breast and prostate cancer deaths despite being hindered with severe obesity and the largest burden of smokers over age fifty of any western nation.
- Americans have the most successful, most available treatments for chronic diseases like high blood pressure and high cholesterol.
- Americans have the shortest wait times for life-changing surgeries, like cataract and hip replacements, that may not increase survival but greatly impact quality of life.
- Americans have the best access to the newest, most effective drugs.
- Americans have the quickest access to the safest, most advanced medical technologies.
- Americans have the easiest access to specialty doctors, doctors of their choice, doctors who lead the world in health care innovation, regardless of what metrics are used in assessing the sources of medical innovation.

Despite that, most Americans want reforms to bring costs down if quality and choice can be maintained. And reforms could have been achieved without jeopardizing the superior medical care Americans receive right now. After all, the vast majority of Americans already report being very satisfied with their health care system. The would-be reformers could have built on this record with important changes such as breaking down anti-competitive barriers, reducing administrative waste, eliminating mandate-created distortions of the health insurance market, implementing creative tax reforms, introducing reasonable reforms to a medico-legal liability system run amok, and forcing doctors and hospitals to post prices, qualifications, and outcomes—information that is essential to value-based purchasing and fundamental for stimulating competition. Such genuine reforms would have brought down the cost of insurance, reduced the number of uninsured, increased individual choice, and allowed Americans to make value-based decisions for their families. They would have left Americans free to keep their health insurance, retain their chosen doctor, and manage their own and their family's pursuit of medical care without government control.

Entitlement has been a central theme of the Obama administration, whether referring to expanding existing government programs, or wealth redistribution, or creating new social programs paid for by the American taxpayer. The great irony in the Obama administration's latest expansion of entitlements—a trillion dollar commitment of taxpayer money to government controlled health care—is that the administration and the Democrats in Congress have created an entitlement that most Americans don't want. Poll after poll demonstrated that a majority of Americans opposed the Democrats' radical change to America's health care system, not just because of its cost, but because of the specific changes that shift power and control away from the individual and to the federal government, yet the president and congressional Democrats pressed ahead. How quickly they forgot. Americans already soundly rejected gatekeepers limiting access in our disastrous experiment with managed care in the 1990s. The backlash against that grand failure should be a strong reminder of what Americans value. Yet our government refused to listen to its citizens.

Under ObamaCare, many Americans will certainly lose their current insurance and thus access to their chosen doctors. Doctors, too, will be swept up in the coming conflict. While our elected government marches down the path of forcing doctors to swallow government-dictated low reimbursements, surely more and more physicians will refuse to see patients. It is not unimaginable that federal government will soon tie medical licensure to accepting the new edicts, as is already contemplated in Massachusetts, where medical licensure may be tied to accepting the state insurance plan. And it seems likely to many that a lame duck Congress might even put forth a government-run "public option"—an option that shifts huge numbers of privately insured Americans to the burden of an already unsustainable taxpayer-funded entitlement program that ultimately eliminates private insurance choices. Such a public option would interpose bureaucrats between doctors and patients and further restrict access to new drugs, to innovative new cures, and to choice of doctors—effects already proven by our own state-based experiments and in other countries. While Congress and the Obama administration claim otherwise, with a public option costs to the taxpayer increase, and choice and access disappear.

In this volume, health policy experts from the United States, Canada, and Western Europe discuss both what can be expected from the health reform legislation and what alternatives should still be considered. Meanwhile, the questions are many about what opposition can do when governmental power is seized despite the will of the people. At the time of this writing, the consequences of the health care changes are yet to unfold. Many of the important aspects of the legislation do not begin until 2014, so the electorate can still be heard. Legal battles questioning the constitutionality of the legislation are already underway in many states; political activists are targeting the rogue politicians who flaunted their own agenda in the face of the constituents who elected them in the first place. The health care debate has become front and center and is certain to remain there for some time.

Now is the time for all who value control of their own health decisions, access to highly trained doctors of their own choosing, continued innovation in new diagnostic methods, and safer, more effective treatments to recognize what they are about to lose. Now is the time to elect leaders who recognize that government control cannot reduce health care costs without restricting choice and access of individuals. Our government can be a positive piece of the health care puzzle by facilitating competitive markets, marketplaces that provide more choices, better care, higher quality, and cost based on value. At this critical juncture,

America needs bold political leaders to stop the inexorable slide to the European social democracy model embracing nationalized health care. If the Congress enacts reforms that remove artificial barriers and constructively open markets to competition, private sector creativity will generate innovative, low-cost insurance products for tens of millions of newly empowered value-conscious shoppers. Innovation comes from the private sector, not government, and there is no reason the health care industry would be an exception. Under ObamaCare, American health care is at serious risk, and that is one government entitlement that we absolutely cannot afford.

—Scott W. Atlas, MD

AMERICAN HEALTH CARE: IGNORED FACTS AND DISREGARDED OPTIONS

Scott W. Atlas, MD

M EDICAL CARE in the United States has been loudly derided as inferior in comparison to health care systems in the rest of the developed world in highly publicized rankings, most notably the World Health Organization's World Health Report comparing health care in almost two hundred nations. These rankings have gained tremendous traction, despite being exposed in leading academic journals for gross distortions from severe methodological flaws, including huge measurement errors that produce results with no statistical significance, data missing from dozens of countries, biased assumptions, and extreme subjectivity.[1] Government officials, policymakers, insurers and even many academics used this pseudo-data to justify their personal agenda centralizing power over health care to government by imposing the

---

Scott Atlas is a senior fellow at the Hoover Institution and professor at Stanford University Medical Center. He can be reached at swatlas@stanford.edu.

radical changes to America's health care contained in the Patient Protection and Affordable Care Act (also known as "ObamaCare") on a largely unwilling public.

Why has the public remained steadfast in its opposition to the reforms imposed by Congress and President Obama? On one hand, much of the American public still assumes the criticisms of our system are sound, because the calls for change have been so ubiquitous and the topic so complex. Indeed, a large majority of Americans have repeatedly concurred that their health care system needs "fundamental change" or "complete rebuilding."[2] Yet despite that general opinion, in multiple studies, over 80 percent of Americans are satisfied with the quality of their own health care, a number rising steadily over the past several years.[3] (This striking contradiction in public opinion, while ignored by policymakers calling for radical changes in the debate over the state of America's health care, reveals the fundamental truth: Americans understand, from personal experience, that American medical care is the best in the world. Americans understand what they could lose in a government-centralized health system in which government is empowered to exercise unprecedented control over the most personal decisions in the lives of individuals.

IGNORED FACTS: AMERICAN HEALTH CARE IS SUPERIOR

The reality, from analysis of facts, is that American health care is superior. This inescapable conclusion derives from actual data, not opinion. The world's leading journals are filled with studies demonstrating the superiority of American medical care to care found in other countries with systems more heavily controlled by government bodies. These studies verify better survival from serious diseases like cancer, better access to treatment for the most prevalent chronic diseases, wider access to preventive care and cancer screening, broader availability of the newest life-changing medical technology, wider access to the most accurate diagnostic technology, quicker access to innovative, life-saving cures and safer, less invasive treatments, more rapid access to highly trained specialists, and ultimately far better access to the world's leading doctors and medical scientists who themselves are the source of the world's leading innovations by any metric examined.

Before accepting a radical overhaul of the world's leading medical care system, and instead of turning to government as the solution to the widely recognized problems of health care, these important unheralded facts about America's health care system should be carefully considered.

Fact No. 1: Americans have better survival rates than Europeans for most common as well as rare cancers.[4] (See Figure 1.1.) Among more common cancers, the breast cancer mortality rate is 52 percent higher in Germany than in the United States, and 88 percent higher in the United Kingdom. Prostate cancer mortality is strikingly higher in the UK and in Norway. Age-standardized death rates from prostate cancer from 1980–2005 have been reduced far faster in the United States than in the fifteen other developed nations studied, attesting to superior outcomes in

FIGURE 1.1
Five-year cancer survival rates, %

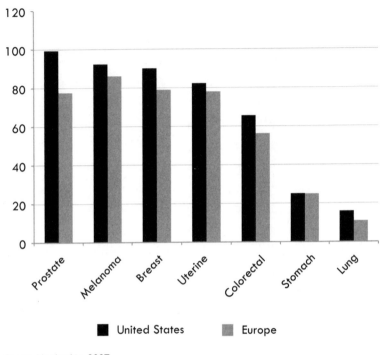

■ United States   ■ Europe

Source: Verdecchio, 2007

what is the most common cancer among men.[5] The mortality rate for colorectal cancer among British men and women is about 40 percent higher. Americans, whether men or women, enjoy superior overall survival from cancer than western Europeans. (See Figure 1.2.)

Fact No. 2: Americans have lower cancer mortality rates than Canadians.[6] Breast cancer mortality is 9 percent higher, for example; prostate cancer is 184 percent higher; and colon cancer mortality among men is about 10 percent higher than in the United States.

FIGURE 1.2
Five-year cancer survival rates, %

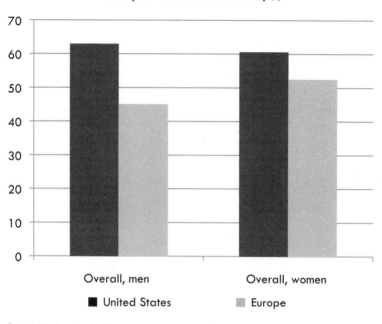

Source: Verdecchio, 2007

Fact No. 3: Americans have better access to treatment for chronic diseases than patients in other developed countries.[7] Some 56 percent of Americans who could benefit are taking statins, which reduce cholesterol and protect against heart disease. By comparison, of those patients who could benefit from these drugs, only 36 percent of the Dutch, 29 percent of the Swiss, 26 percent of Germans, 23 percent of Britons, and 17 percent of Italians receive them.

Fact No. 4: Americans have better access to preventive cancer screening than Canadians.[8] Take the proportion of the appropriate-age population groups who have received recommended tests for breast, cervical, prostrate and colon cancer:

- Nine out of ten middle-aged American women (89 percent) have had a mammogram, compared to less than three-fourths of Canadians (72 percent).
- Nearly all American women (96 percent) have had a pap smear, compared to less than 90 percent of Canadians.
- More than half of U.S. men (54 percent) have had a PSA test, compared to less than 1 in 6 Canadians (16 percent).
- Nearly one-third of Americans (30 percent) have had a colonoscopy, compared with less than 1 in 20 Canadians (5 percent).

Fact No. 5: Lower-income Americans are in better health than comparable Canadians. It is often claimed that government-financed health care systems, such as Canada's, eliminate income-related barriers to health. The "health-income gradient" (i.e. the concept that higher income achieves better health, and lower income means worse health) for adults 16 to 64 years old reveals a more severe disparity in Canada than in the United States. Specifically, twice as many American seniors with below-median incomes self-report "excellent" health compared to Canadian seniors (11.7 percent versus 5.8 percent). Conversely, white Canadian young adults with below-median incomes are 20 percent more likely than lower-income Americans to describe their health as "fair or poor."[9]

Fact No. 6: Americans spend much less time waiting than patients in Canada and the UK—to see a specialist,

to have life-changing elective surgery like hip replacements or cataract removal, or to get radiation treatment for cancer.[10] All told, 827,429 people are waiting for some type of procedure in Canada.[11] In England, nearly 1.8 million people are waiting for a hospital admission or outpatient treatment.[12]

Fact No. 7: Americans are not alone, among residents of developed countries, in believing their health systems need major reforms. The unspoken truth is that those with more government control of their health systems, the very countries purported to serve as the models for a reformed American system, are similarly highly dissatisfied and believe their own health systems need fundamental change or complete rebuilding. (See Figure 1.3.) More than 70 percent of German, Canadian, Australian, New Zealand and British adults, say their health systems need either "fundamental change" or "complete rebuilding,"[13] and 60 percent of western Europeans say their systems need "urgent" reform.[14]

Fact No. 8: Americans are more satisfied with the care they receive than Canadians, a highly government-controlled health system often portrayed by the media as a system to emulate. When asked directly about their own health care instead of the "health care system," more than half of Americans (51.3 percent) are very satisfied with their health care services, compared to only 41.5 percent of Canadians; fewer Americans are dissatisfied (6.8 percent) than Canadians (8.5 percent).[15]

Fact No. 9: Americans have much better access to important new technologies like medical imaging than patients in Canada or the UK. An overwhelming majority

FIGURE 1.3

Other Developed Countries: Models for Health System Satisfaction
What reform is needed

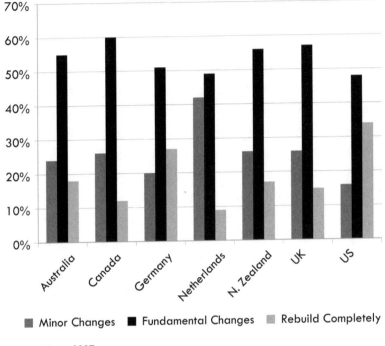

■ Minor Changes   ■ Fundamental Changes   ▨ Rebuild Completely

Source: Schoen, 2007

of leading American physicians say computerized tomogra-
phy (CT) and magnetic resonance imaging (MRI), which
have been maligned as a waste by economists and targeted
by the Congress and many policymakers naïve to actual
medical practice, were the most important medical innovations for improving patient care during the previous decade.[16] The United States has thirty-four CT scanners per
million population, compared to twelve in Canada and

eight in Britain. The United States has nearly twenty-seven MRI machines per million compared to about six per million in Canada and Britain.[17]

Fact No. 10: By any variety of measures, Americans are responsible for the vast majority of all health care innovations, innovations from which the entire world benefits.[18] The top five U.S. hospitals conduct more clinical trials than all the hospitals in any other single developed country.[19] Since the mid-1970s, the Nobel Prize in medicine or physiology has gone to American residents more often than recipients from all other countries combined.[20] (See Figure 1.4.) From 1969 to 2008, Americans (2009 population 307 million) won or shared the Nobel Prize in Medicine and Physiology fifty-seven times compared with forty times by medical scientists from the European Union, Switzerland, Japan, Canada, and Australia combined (2009 population 681 million).[21] Indeed, of the past thirty-four years, there were only five years in which a scientist living in America didn't either win or share in the prize.

DISREGARDED OPTIONS: INDIVIDUAL EMPOWERMENT NOT GOVERNMENT CENTRALIZATION

Regardless of the amazing quality of medical care that has evolved over the past half century and even acknowledging that the U.S. health care system compares favorably to those in other developed countries, there is a broad consensus on a number of significant problems in American health care. It is inarguable that costs are high and increasing. It is also

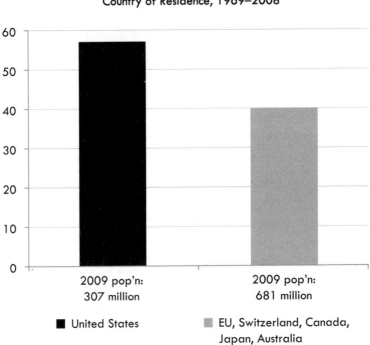

FIGURE 1.4
Nobel Prizes in Medicine and Physiology by
Country of Residence, 1969–2008

■ United States   EU, Switzerland, Canada,
                           Japan, Australia

Source: Whitman and Raad, 2009; Bending the Productivity Curve:
Why America Leads the World in Medical Innovation

clear that government and society cannot continue to spend such huge sums of money and large proportion of GDP on health care. The lack of portability of health insurance in the American system, which largely relies on employers for insurance, needs to be changed. The fact that millions of Americans are uninsured must be addressed.

The Democrat Congress and the Obama administration claim that a major principle underlying their health reform law rests on the goal of increasing competition among health insurance providers. Increasing competition would seem to be a fundamental means of reducing cost, but to the contrary the new legislation will only centralize power to the government. The health legislation passed by the Congress and the Obama administration creates massive new government authority that controls access to medical care and insurance benefits. Rather than increasing private sector competition, the legislation will reduce choice, shift more regulatory power to bureaucrats, hinder innovation, and ultimately be likely to serve as a rationale for shifting Americans to public plans that restrict access to care.

The overall goal of any health reform plan should be to increase the opportunity for good health for Americans and their families. Key principles include reducing the number of uninsured, facilitating access to affordable health insurance, making health insurance more portable, and promoting innovation in health care, so that the excellence of American health care is not sacrificed and individuals and their families are empowered to decide how best to spend their money in health care decisions. Here are six straightforward steps the government could take, right now, that would increase the competitiveness in the health insurance markets and empower consumers so costs come down by value-based purchasing rather than government edict. These reforms will reduce the number of uninsured, facilitate access to affordable insurance, make health insurance portable, and promote innovation in health care.

A first step to increasing competitiveness in the health insurance market is to allow cross-state purchasing, so that people can shop at competitive prices in a national market for the insurance they actually want to buy. It is ill-conceived, unnecessary, and self-defeating to the goal of encouraging competition that Americans are forced to restrict their purchases to in-state goods or services. Government can rapidly lower the price of health insurance through the private insurance market by breaking down these anti-competitive barriers that result in shocking variations on the order of several multiples among states in prices for equivalent health coverage. One specific and immediate action would be to allow small businesses to band together in trade associations to purchase coverage for their employees. If regulated by the Employee Retirement Income Security Act of 1974 (ERISA), they would be exempt from state health insurance mandates and regulations. Just like large businesses, America's small businesses need this capacity now, so their employees can save money by getting the coverage they actually want instead of bloated plans they don't desire. Since small business employees make up the biggest proportion of uninsured workers, this one change would have high impact.

Second, government can force transparency on the system, ensuring that Americans have a clear understanding of the price and quality of their doctors and hospitals, as well as enough information about health and diseases to make informed, value-conscious decisions. Let's leave the experts—medical scientists in their peer-reviewed literature—to determine efficacy and clinical utility. A far more important role of the government needs to be explored: to make transparent the pricing of medical procedures. Public knowledge of price will provide an important impetus toward competitive pricing by both physicians and hospitals. In our current system, few patients are aware of the charges about to be incurred for their medical care. Generally, they have no reason to ask because the current third-party-payer structure makes patients believe that "someone else is paying." The lack of patient demand for price information has allowed hospitals and doctors to cloak their price structure in a shroud of mystery and avoid public view. A powerful role of the government could be to require posting of prices for medical procedures and services, as well as qualifications of doctors. Information is power, and price visibility is essential to induce competition.

Third, it is time to reduce the mandate-created distortions of health insurance markets. State-based mandates alone now number over 2,100 and are a scandalous abuse of government dictates. They increase insurance costs by 20 to 50 percent, and force Americans to buy policies covering massage therapy, acupuncture, chiropractors, *in vitro* fertilization, wigs, and other services not necessarily wanted by more than a small minority of American families. Instead of adding mandates to purchase insurance that Americans rationally do not consider a good value, the government should instead focus on creating an environment where insurance products can become attractive to consumers. Governments can put a halt to the unending stream of expensive coverage mandates advocated by special interest groups and intrusive big government supporters and start stripping back on these costly and ill-advised regulations.

The fact is that the problems with our system today are to a great extent caused by decades of failed and costly government mandates, and the huge burden of government intrusion into our health care decisions. For a president and a party who voice concern about the right to privacy, it seems paradoxical to push government into such personal decisions as medical care. How about letting patients themselves decide what sort of coverage and benefits they want for their families by watching what they actually purchase, rather than defining appropriate coverage as if they were naïve children or simply incompetent?

Fourth, it's sensible to expand consumer choice by increasing instead of restricting the availability of insurance and simplifying rather than complicating the rules and regulations of lower-cost health plans, like high deductible plans for catastrophic coverage with health savings accounts. This will make insurance an attractive purchase—a good value—for the millions of Americans who can afford insurance but currently (and arguably wisely) choose to forego buying something they consider a poor value for their money. HSAs increase choice for consumers, expand individual ownership and control over health spending, promote price visibility to allow value-based purchasing, and provide incentives for savings to prepare for future health care needs. Congress should permit more flexibility in employer contributions to "disease management accounts" in lieu of traditional third-party benefits, support tax reform proposals to allow parents' HSA balances to transfer to their children's HSAs tax-free, and allow holders of HSA plans who relocate because of a job change to purchase health insurance across state lines without being subject to state mandates.

Fifth, government can empower the consumer, instead of itself, by revamping the tax treatment of health care expenses, so that all Americans will truly shop for and ultimately own their health insurance. A number of creative reforms have gone ignored by those more interested in empowering government rather than American families with control of the money. For instance, a national system of refundable health care tax credits—actual cash even for those who pay no income tax—would foster personal ownership and control of health plans and increase the market competition that the administration claims it seeks to advance. The essential portability of insurance—truly owned and designed by American consumers—eliminates the fear of job loss and exposure to financial disaster by loss of coverage and creates a huge new group of value-seeking shoppers for insurance. Instead of expanding dependence on the already unsustainable government health plans of Medicare and Medicaid and then reducing payments that restrict medical care, vouchers can partly or even totally replace those systems, creating a massive new market of Americans shopping for personally valued insurance from a responsive private sector. Innovation comes from the private sector, not government, and there is no reason the health insurance industry would be an exception if the appropriate incentives and opportunities were put in place. Moreover, the illusion that private insurers are evil and government insurance is somehow more benevolent is exposed by facts showing that Medicare has the highest rate of claim denials, 6.85 percent, compared with all seven private insurance companies.[22] Empowerment means having control of the health care dollar, and with it, decision-making authority over medical care and doctor selection, insurance coverage people want rather than are forced to pay for, and coverage that is affordable and portable. This single policy change would reduce health expenditures on the order of hundreds of billions of dollars, while simultaneously eliminating the crippling burden of health costs on American businesses created by historical accident rather than thoughtful intention.

Sixth, Congress can finally have the courage to push back against the trial lawyers and fix the medical liability system. Even acknowledging the important goals of ensuring quality and protecting patients' rights, the medical-liability legal system imposes a tremendous financial burden on the health care system in the United States, estimated at over 80 billion dollars per year. Doctors and hospitals not only pass on the direct costs of increased malpractice premiums, but provide more expensive and relatively unproductive medical treatments out of fear of litigation. Estimates are that the additional cost of defensive medicine can amount to tens of billions of dollars per year, up to 6 percent of total costs. A significant rethinking of the entire legal relationship between patient and care provider needs to be considered. Even in advance of that, research by academics and government agencies is clear: common sense reforms to the medical liability system, like reasonable caps on non-economic damages and giving patients and providers more freedom to experiment with alternatives to traditional courts for resolving disputes, can compensate victims more quickly, reduce costs, and enhance incentives for doctors and hospitals to take more appropriate precautions against medical errors.

CONCLUSION

While our elected senators and representatives, under the direction of the Obama administration, debated their ideas to wholly reconfigure America's health care system at a massive cost to our children and future generations, they continued to deny that clear alternative reforms exist to lower health care costs, increase choice of insurance, and maintain the excellence of our medical system. Cloaked with the straw man argument that "doing nothing is simply unacceptable," our government embarked on a sweeping takeover of America's health care. Finally, the Democratic Congress voted for a 2,500-page bill that pushes a radical overhaul of the world's most advanced health care, a bill opposed by the majority of American voters, and paid at a cost of a trillion dollars by massive taxes, penalties, and cuts in coverage. That legislation is based on government mandates and penalties on individuals and businesses, a dramatic expansion of already unsustainable government insurance programs, and new government authority to regulate access to medical care, physician-patient decision-making autonomy, and insurance benefits.

It may shock many Americans that the same health systems held up as models by those interested in overhauling

America's are held in very poor regard by the very people who live under them. Meanwhile, evidence shows that countries with heavy-handed government-run health care have failed to control escalating costs. Even welfare-burdened nations like Sweden are introducing privatization as part of their solution in grappling with the economic challenges of health care. Consider that 80 percent of Americans say that access to the most advanced tests, drugs, and medical procedures and equipment is "very important" or "absolutely essential" yet our government's economic advisors stress limiting their use. And why is it that those government officials leading the charge toward nationalized health care immediately wield all their influence to seek out America's leading physicians and the most sophisticated diagnostic tests and novel therapies behind closed doors, when they or their families need care? Ironically, they themselves should be particularly worried, because ultimately we risk an inevitable degradation of physician quality, owing to the impending price (and therefore wage) controls for health care providers and hospitals. Does anyone really believe that the best and brightest will continue to pursue a profession requiring years of rigorous training and sacrifice when in the end government fixes wages and bureaucrats dictate decisions? And does anyone really think that the federal government will not eventually try to force doctors to accept new low prices by threatening additional licensure requirements based on acceptance of those prices, a shift of authority to big brother government that is already proposed in Massachusetts?

Ironically, much of the urgency for reform was pressed on the American people by distorting the problems with the system and blatantly ignoring the facts that point to the excellence, and indeed the superiority, of American medical care. While the economic failures of the growing health care expenditure burden are enormous and fearful to contemplate on a national scale, it may be that the more dangerous consequences of the impending radical transformation of America's health care system will be far more personal to Americans and their families. With all its flaws, the leadership position of American health care is at serious risk. Americans enjoy unrivalled access to the most advanced medical care in the world, and important facts—data published in leading peer-reviewed journals—point to the superiority of America's health care. Now is the time for all who value control of their own health decisions, access to highly trained sub-specialty doctors of their own choosing, continued advances in new diagnostic methods, and safer, more effective treatments to recognize what they are about to lose. We need creative and bold leadership to stop the inexorable slide to nationalization of health care that has been proven world-wide to reduce choice, restrict access, and harm patient outcomes. The shift of power from patients and their doctors to government bureaucrats under the guise of reducing costs may be the greatest Trojan horse in American history. If allowed to stand, this would mark the end of health care as we know it.

NOTES

1. C. Almeida, P. Braveman et al. "Methodological Concerns and Recommendations on Policy Consequences of the World Health Report

2000." *Lancet* 357 (2001): 1692–7; Y. Asada and T. Hedemann "A Problem with the Individual Approach in the WHO Inequality Measurement," *International Journal for Equity in Health* 1:2 (2002); P. Musgrove, "Judging Health Systems: Reflections on WHO's Methods." *Lancet* 361 (2003): 1817; V. Navarro, Assessment of the World Health Report 2000. *Lancet* 356 (2000); 1598–1601; E. Ollila and M. Koivusalo, "The World Health Report 2000: World Health Organization Health Policy Steering Off Course—Change Values, Poor Evidence, and Lack of Accountability." *International Journal of Health Services* 32 (2002): 503–514; G. Whitman, "WHO's Fooling Who? The World Health Organization's Problematic Ranking of Health Care Systems," Cato Institute, Briefing 101, February 28, 2008.

2. Cathy Schoen et al, "Toward Higher Performance Health Systems: Adults' Health Care Experiences in Seven Countries;" *Health Affairs* 26 (2007): w717–734; CBS/*NewYork Times* poll, April 2009.

3. CNN/Opinion Research Corp poll, March 2009; Gallup polls 2007, 2006, 2005, 2004, 2003, 2002, 2001; Quinnipiac University poll, October 2007; etc.

4. Concord Working Group, "Cancer Survival in Five Continents: A Worldwide Population-based Study," *Lancet Oncology*, 9, no. 8 (2008): 730–756; Arduino Verdecchia et al., "Recent Cancer Survival in Europe: A 2000–02 Period Analysis of EUROCARE-4 Data," *Lancet Oncology*, 8, no. 9, (2007): 784–796; *Lancet Oncology* 7, no. 2 (2006): 132–140.

5. Samuel H. Preston and Jessica Ho, "Low Life Expectancy in the United States: Is the Health Care System at Fault?" PSC Working Paper Series, PSC 09–03 (2009).

6. U.S. Cancer Statistics, National Program of Cancer Registries, U.S. Centers for Disease Control; Canadian Cancer Society/National Cancer Institute of Canada; see also June O'Neill and Dave M. O'Neill, "Health Status, Health Care and Inequality: Canada vs. the U.S.," National Bureau of Economic Research, Working Paper No. 13429 (September 2007). Available at www.nber.org/papers/w13429.

7. Oliver Schoffski (University of Erlangen-Nuremberg), "Diffusion of Medicines in Europe," European Federation of Pharmaceutical Industries and Associations (2002). Available at www.amchampc.org/showFile.asp?FID=126. See also Michael Tanner, "The Grass is

Not Always Greener: A Look at National Health Care Systems around the World," Cato Institute, *Policy Analysis* 613 (March 18, 2008); June O'Neill and Dave M. O'Neill, "Health Status, Health Care and Inequality: Canada vs. the U.S.," National Bureau of Economic Research, NBER Working Paper 13429 (September 2007).

8. June O'Neill and Dave M. O'Neill, "Health Status, Health Care and Inequality: Canada vs. the U.S."

9. Ibid.

10. Nadeem Esmail, Michael A. Walker with Margaret Bank, "Waiting Your Turn (17th edition): Hospital Waiting Lists In Canada," Fraser Institute, Critical Issues Bulletin 2007, Studies in Health Care Policy (August 2008); Nadeem Esmail and Dominika Wrona "Medical Technology in Canada," Fraser Institute (August 21, 2008); Sharon Willcox et al., "Measuring and Reducing Waiting Times: A Cross-National Comparison Of Strategies," *Health Affairs* 26, no. 4 (July/August 2007) 1,078–87; June O'Neill and Dave M. O'Neill, "Health Status, Health Care and Inequality: Canada vs. the U.S."; M. V. Williams et al., "Radiotherapy Dose Fractionation, Access and Waiting Times in the Countries of the U.K. in 2005," Royal College of Radiologists, *Clinical Oncology*,19, no. 5 (June 2007) 273–286.

11. Nadeem Esmail and Michael A. Walker with Margaret Bank, "Waiting Your Turn (17th Edition): Hospital Waiting Lists In Canada 2007."

12. "Hospital Waiting Times and List Statistics," Department of Health, England. Available at www.dh.gov.uk/en/Publicationsand statistics/Statistics/Performancedataandstatistics/HospitalWaiting TimesandListStatistics/index.htm?IdcService=GET_FILE&dID=186979 &Rendition=Web.

13. Cathy Schoen et al., "Toward Higher-Performance Health Systems: Adults' Health Care Experiences In Seven Countries, 2007," *Health Affairs*, Web Exclusive 26, no. 6 (October 31, 2007) w717–w734. Available at http://content.healthaffairs.org/cgi/reprint/26/6/w717.

14. "Impatient for Change: European Attitudes to Healthcare Reform;" The Stockholm Network (2004); H. Disney et al.

15. June O'Neill and Dave M. O'Neill, "Health Status, Health Care and Inequality: Canada vs. the U.S."

16. Victor R. Fuchs and Harold C. Sox Jr., "Physicians' Views of the Relative Importance of 30 Medical Innovations," *Health Affairs* 20, no. 5 (September/October 2001) 30–42. Available at http://content .healthaffairs.org/cgi/reprint/20/5/30.pdf.

17. OECD Health Data 2008, Organization for Economic Cooperation and Development. Available at www.oecd.org/document/30/ 0,3343,en_2649_34631_12968734_1_1_1_37407,00.html.

18. "The U.S. Health Care System as an Engine of Innovation," *Economic Report of the President* Washington, DC: Government Printing Office, 2004, 108th Congress, 2nd Session H. Doc. 108–145, Chapter 10, 190–193, available at www.gpoaccess.gov/usbudget/fy05/pdf/2004 _erp.pdf; Tyler Cowen, *New York Times*, Oct. 5, 2006; Tom Coburn, Joseph Antos and Grace-Marie Turner, "Competition: A Prescription for Health Care Transformation," Heritage Foundation, Lecture No. 1030, April 2007; Thomas Boehm, "How can we explain the American dominance in biomedical research and development?" *Journal of Medical Marketing*, 5, no. 2 (2005) 158–66, U.S. Department of Health and Human Services, July 2002. Available at http://fraser.stlouisfed.org/ publications/erp/page/8649/download/47455/8649_ERP.pdf.

19. Nicholas D. Kristof, "Franklin Delano Obama," *New York Times*, February 28, 2009, available at www.nytimes.com/2009/03/01/opinion/ 01Kristof.html.

20. The Nobel Prize Internet Archive. Available at http://almaz.com/ nobel/medicine/medicine.html.

21. From G. Whitman and Raad, 2009; "Bending the Productivity Curve: Why America Leads the World in Medical Innovation," Cato Institute, Policy Analysis 654 (2009).

22. AMA National Health Insurer Report Card, 2008

2

INDIVIDUAL INSURANCE MANDATES

Glen Whitman

D URING THE 2008 presidential campaign, Barack Obama and Hillary Clinton did battle with competing health care reform plans. Clinton's plan featured an *individual mandate*—that is, a requirement for all Americans to obtain health insurance coverage, whether through an employer, the individual insurance market, or a public plan such as Medicare or Medicaid. Obama denounced the Clinton plan in no uncertain terms:

> A mandate means that, in some fashion, everybody will be forced to buy health insurance ... [T]hat may mean taking money out of people's paychecks in order to make sure that they're covered. . . . The problem is not that folks are trying to avoid getting health care; the problem is they can't afford it.[1]

Upon arrival in the Oval Office, however, Obama reversed course. "I am now in favor of some sort of individual

---

Glen Whitman is professor of economics at California State University, Northridge, and adjunct scholar with the Cato Institute.

mandate as long as there's a hardship exemption," he said in 2009.[2] The individual mandate became a key component in the Patient Protection and Affordable Care Act (PPACA) that he championed and signed into law in March 2010.

President Obama is not alone. Even some people who normally favor free markets[3] have supported some form of an individual mandate.

What makes the individual mandate so seductive that even some of its most vigorous opponents eventually come around? After all, it is not inherently attractive. It forces people to buy something they may not wish to buy, and the resulting financial burden can put heavy stress on already tight household budgets. Arguably, the individual mandate is just a tax—one that flows directly from taxpayers to recipients without going through the public treasury. It reeks of politically guaranteed business for unpopular health insurance companies. Who could support that?

The individual mandate is a mistake—one that will likely cause far greater problems than it solves. It will do nothing to lower health costs and much to drive them ever higher. But to understand what's wrong with the mandate, we need to understand its appeal. For the most part, advocates support the individual mandate as a *patch* for problems created by other regulations of the health insurance market.

ADVERSE SELECTION AND INSURANCE REGULATION

The most frequently cited justification for the individual mandate is to encourage pooling of risk, thereby avoiding the problem of adverse selection.

Adverse selection is a problem that can afflict insurance markets when potential policy buyers have different expected costs. In general, any given premium will be most desirable to people with higher expected costs, such as the elderly and people with pre-existing medical conditions. Meanwhile, the premium will seem unreasonably high to those with lower expected costs, usually younger people. Some of the latter group may therefore choose to go uninsured. As a result, the insurance company ends up with a pool of higher-cost patients and therefore has to raise premiums. Those higher premiums may trigger another round of patients to choose to go uninsured—and so on. The process is called "adverse" because it tends to result in disproportionate numbers of high-cost patients relative to low-cost patients getting insured.

You can find a description of the adverse selection problem in most intermediate economics textbooks, not to mention numerous reports and studies on health care policy. (The 2010 Economic Report of the President is just one example.[4]) These descriptions often fail to mention, however, that adverse selection is largely a *solved problem*. Insurance markets have well-established means of keeping adverse selection in check.

The most important such method is charging premiums based on risk—what is known in the industry as *underwriting*. This method is widely accepted in auto insurance markets, where people with worse driving records and longer commutes have to pay more for their coverage. Drivers with lower expected costs pay less; drivers with higher expected costs pay more. Nobody thinks the purpose of auto insurance is to make good drivers pay for the accidents of bad drivers.

But in the health insurance market, underwriting is often looked upon with anger and suspicion. As a result, it attracts regulation. One popular form of regulation is *community rating*, which prohibits insurance companies from charging different premiums to people within the same community based on health-related factors. (Community rating comes in different forms; sometimes it allows premium differentials based on age and gender, for instance.) Community rating exacerbates the adverse selection problem. When people with different levels of expected cost face the same or similar premiums, the lower-cost people are more likely to choose to go uninsured.

Another popular form of regulation is *guaranteed issue*, which requires insurance companies to offer coverage to anyone in their region. The purpose, among other things, is to prevent the rejection of people with pre-existing conditions. Although insurance companies could comply by offering coverage at prohibitively high premiums, guaranteed issue is typically accompanied by other regulations—such as community rating—to make sure policies are offered to everyone at similar rates.

Guaranteed issue aggravates the adverse selection problem by opening the door to opportunistic behavior. Imagine if you could buy auto insurance *after* having an accident; would you bother to carry insurance? When people know they can get insurance whenever they need it, they can simply wait until they get sick. And this perverse incentive potentially affects everybody, not just the young and healthy. Insurance companies, in response, must raise premiums to cover the disproportionate number of sick people they cover.

Community rating, guaranteed issue, and other related regulations are usually well-intentioned. They aim to make affordable coverage available to everyone. But in reality, they create unintended consequences. They drive up premiums, thereby pushing some people—especially the young, healthy, and poor—into the ranks of the uninsured.

The 2010 health care legislation takes community rating and guaranteed issue, which previously were implemented only at the state level, and federalizes them. The new law prohibits underwriting based on "health status, mental or physical medical conditions, claims experience, medical history, genetic information, disability, other evidence of insurability, or other factors to be determined later by the secretary of HHS."[5] The only factors insurers may consider under the law are age, smoking status, and geography. Even the age differentials will be limited to a three-to-one ratio across age groups; that is, the premium for an older patient may not exceed three times the premium for a younger (but otherwise similar) patient.[6]

According to a Rand Corporation study, premiums for people under the age of 35 can be expected to rise by 17 percent as a result of the law's community rating regulation.[7] That figure is actually a low-end estimate on expected premium hikes for lower-cost buyers because the Rand study considered only the restriction on age-based pricing and not the law's other underwriting restrictions. Faced with substantial premium hikes, many young and healthy people might prefer to opt out.

And that is why the new law includes an individual mandate. Since adverse selection results from some individuals choosing not to buy insurance when premiums are too high, the hope is that forcing everyone to buy will make the problem go away. The Economic Report of the President, for instance, argued: "To prevent a spiral of increasing costs and decreasing insurance rates resulting from adverse selection, both the House and the Senate bills establish a principle of joint individual and employer responsibility to obtain and provide insurance, and would provide subsidies and tax credits that would assist in this process."[8] In the end, that argument carried the day.

FREE RIDERS AND THE SAMARITANS' DILEMMA

Adverse selection is not the only justification offered for the individual mandate. Some supporters—particularly those who usually favor free markets—reluctantly support an individual mandate in order to deal with the *free-rider problem* associated with uncompensated care.

People without health insurance don't necessarily go without care. They still arrive in medical facilities, particularly emergency rooms, and providers are often unable or unwilling to turn them away. In some cases, providers are legally or ethically obliged to provide care. The cost of that care is—one way or another—paid by the rest of us.

The result is sometimes called the Samaritans' Dilemma: precisely because of our compassion, we can be taken advantage of. Some people who could in principle afford health insurance may opt out, knowing the system will still take care of them. This concern is particularly salient when taxpayers are expected to pay, as in the case of public emergency rooms.[9]

But how serious is the free-riding problem? According to the Economic Report of the President, total uncompensated health expenditures in 2008 amounted to $56 billion.[10] That sounds like a lot, until you realize that total health expenditures in that year were $2.3 trillion.[11] Thus, uncompensated care accounted for only 2.4 percent of all health expenditures. Not surprisingly, uninsured people tend to make less use of the health care system. If you want to know why U.S. health care is expensive, look elsewhere.

Furthermore, lack of insurance and free-riding are not synonymous. There are other ways to pay for treatment; it turns out that uninsured people pay out of pocket for about 25 percent of their health expenditures. And conversely, having insurance doesn't mean all your care is covered; about 30 percent of all uncompensated care is for insured patients (such as those who don't pay their co-payments).[12] So even if an individual mandate meant everyone would be insured, uncompensated care would still be an issue.

The figures for uncompensated care do not include care paid for by public aid programs, such as Medicare and Medicaid, which count as forms of insurance coverage. The taxpaying public foots the bill for a much larger fraction of health spending than 2.4 percent. But nobody expects an individual mandate to reduce those public expenditures. On the contrary, it is widely recognized that the individual mandate will fail without extensive subsidies for those unable to afford coverage. The new health care law includes major expansions of both Medicaid and State Children's Health Insurance Program (SCHIP), as well as expanded funding for community health centers and subsidies to small businesses.[13]

A QUESTION OF COMPLIANCE

The efficacy of the individual mandate will depend on how many people comply with the mandate. But as anyone who has ever driven over the speed limit knows, compliance cannot be taken for granted.

Auto insurance is mandatory for drivers in forty-nine states (all but New Hampshire). Yet the percentage of drivers who are uninsured nationwide hovers around 14 percent. In five states, the percentage of drivers who are uninsured exceeds 20 percent.[14]

Of course, the percentage might be even higher without a mandate. The point is that any degree of noncompliance will reduce the expected benefits of a mandate to the same degree.

Although some people will comply simply out of respect for the law, others will only do so if they will be punished otherwise. And even then, the punishment must be dire enough to make purchasing an expensive product—one they have already demonstrated an unwillingness to buy—worthwhile.

The new health care law creates a rising penalty, starting in 2014 at $95 or 1 percent of income (whichever is higher) and rising to $325 or 2 percent of income in 2015.[15] Only time will tell if these penalties are sufficient, but we can speculate. Between an insurance plan costing $3,000 over the year[16] and a payment of $325, which is a low-income individual more likely to choose? Especially given guaranteed issue, which will allow them to purchase later if they become sick, paying the penalty could be a no-brainer.

Massachusetts passed a health reform bill with an individual mandate in 2006. By 2008, the uninsured rate in that state had fallen from 10 percent to approximately 4 percent.[17] Looking at the glass as half-full, the mandate helped to reduce the uninsured rate by more than half. Looking at the glass half-empty, about 40 percent of the targeted population is still not complying with the law.

More worrisome, evidence suggests that some of the new coverage is opportunistic coverage—that is, people taking advantage of guaranteed issue by buying coverage when they get sick and dropping it once they are well. A report issued by the Massachusetts Division of Insurance reports a quadrupling, between 2006 and 2008, of the number of people dropping their insurance within six months of acquiring it.[18]

The Massachusetts law also includes substantial subsidies for the purchase of insurance, which means that the reduction in the number of uninsured cannot be attributed entirely to the individual mandate. Indeed, the greatest increases in coverage took place among those groups targeted by the subsidies; 58 percent of those newly insured had their care paid for by the government.[19] The subsidies were originally projected to cost the state an additional $725 million per year; this estimate was later revised upward to $880 million by the year 2010.[20] It therefore seems probable that subsidies are doing much of the work.

THE MINIMUM BENEFITS PACKAGE

To mandate something, you have to define it. The law needs to specify all features and benefits an insurance policy must have in order to qualify.

Sadly, the benefits package cannot be defined in an apolitical way. There is no objective, scientific way to define a phrase like "medically necessary." Instead, the legislators and bureaucrats empowered to decide bring their own subjective beliefs, judgments, and biases to the table. In the process, they are inevitably influenced by interested parties. The lobbying arms of every medical specialty and profession, from oncology to acupuncture, have a strong incentive to push for their services to be included in the package—and covered generously.

The 2010 health care law already establishes a generous set of minimum benefits. The package includes ambulatory patient services, emergency services, hospitalization, maternity and newborn care, mental health and substance abuse services, prescription drugs, rehabilitative services and devices, laboratory services, preventive care and wellness care, chronic disease management, and pediatric services (including vision and dental care).[21] The law further empowers the Secretary of Health and Human Services to define all these terms.[22]

Both the statute and its accompanying regulations will evolve over time in response to ongoing special-interest pressures. We can therefore expect the universally mandated benefits package to become more bloated over time. As the benefits package grows, so will premiums. With the financial burden of the mandate rising, we may also see more individuals and households deciding noncompliance is the best option. Others will comply only by relying on public subsidies, whose burden will also rise over time.

The political dynamic described here is far from speculative. It has been demonstrated already at the state level. Every state in the union has its own list of legally mandated benefits that every health insurance policy must cover. Some states have mandated coverage of contraception, dental care, chiropractic, in vitro fertilization, and hair transplants, just to name a few. Over 2,100 such laws are on the books—an average of forty-two mandated benefits per state.[23] These are the fruit of lobbying efforts by medical specialties that stand to gain from the increased business.[24] Consumers pay for the mandates with higher insurance premiums, which the mandates drive up by 20 percent or more depending on the state.[25]

Special interests have pushed for state-level mandated benefits even when they apply only to voluntarily purchased policies. When a nationwide benefits package is mandated for all individuals, the incentive for special interests to get involved will be correspondingly massive.

The Massachusetts experience provides some evidence of the premium-inflating effect of the individual mandate. After passage of the individual mandate, average premiums for individuals in Massachusetts rose 7 percent in both 2007 and 2008; for families, 7 percent in 2007 and

8 percent in 2008.[26] Massachusetts, always an expensive state for insurance, now has the highest insurance premiums in the country.[27] In April of 2010, the insurance commission of Massachusetts took the unprecedented step of denying 235 out of 274 rate increases proposed by insurance firms. The firms had requested increases ranging from 7 to 34 percent.[28]

Aside from defining benefits, an individual mandate must also set criteria for other policy features: maximum payouts, deductibles, co-payments, and so on. Higher deductibles and co-payments generally correspond to lower premiums. Although at present the law permits relatively high deductibles of $5,000 for an individual and $10,000 for a family,[29] it also requires that, on average, policyholders cannot pay more than 40 percent of their covered health expenditures out-of-pocket.[30] The latter requirement will probably result in lower maximum deductibles in practice. Furthermore, this is only the starting point, as the law's coinsurance requirements will evolve over time in response to the same political pressures described above. Health care providers have a financial incentive to support lower deductibles and co-payments, thereby encouraging people to consume more services. Again, the likely outcome is higher premiums, greater noncompliance, and heavier reliance on public subsidies.

If we want to reduce health care costs, insurance firms need to be able to experiment with different kinds of insurance contracts—particularly designs that would provide stronger incentives for patients to weigh the costs and benefits of health services, rather than shielding them from all costs. For instance, firms might want to offer plans that provide full coverage only for lower-cost treatments, while requiring patients to cover the additional cost of choosing more expensive treatments. (This is similar to having low co-payments for generic drugs but higher co-payments for name-brand drugs, a common practice now.) Unfortunately, the individual mandate will tend to constrain such innovation, since any new insurance concept will have to satisfy the minimum requirements of the mandate.

SUMMARY

If the individual mandate worked exactly as intended, it still would do nothing to decrease overall health expenditures. It would lower insurance premiums for some (mostly the old and sick) only by raising premiums for others (mostly the young and healthy). In essence, the mandate would simply redistribute wealth from one group to another.

In this sense, the individual mandate constitutes an attempt to transform the health insurance market into a kind of welfare system. If the goal is to help the needy, it would be more honest and transparent to do it the traditional way—by taxing some and subsidizing others—rather than reengineering the insurance market to serve a purpose it was never meant to serve.

In its actual implementation, however, the individual mandate will tend to raise premiums for everyone, not just the young and healthy. This is true for two reasons.

First, imperfect compliance means that the adverse selection problem cannot be abolished. Lower-cost patients will be disproportionately likely to drop out of the system. Guaranteed-issue regulations will exacerbate the problem, as some people will become insured when—and only when—they need the care. As a result, insurance companies will have to raise premiums for everyone else.

Second, the individual mandate forces a one-size-fits-all benefits package on the public, and special-interest politics will cause that package—already generous under present law—to grow over time. Limits on coinsurance will also tend to become more stringent. When the government forces everyone to purchase more generous plans when less generous plans would be more economical, the inevitable result is higher premiums. Those higher premiums will further aggravate the problem of adverse selection. To the extent that people continue to comply with the mandate despite rising premiums, they will increasingly rely on public subsidies to do so.

Given the foregoing objections to the individual mandate, it's reasonable to ask whether there is an alternative to forcing people to buy goods and services they don't wish to buy. The answer is yes. Although proposing a comprehensive health reform package is beyond the scope of this essay, the analysis here suggests an alternative path: rolling back current regulations and allowing insurance markets to operate freely.

If community rating, guaranteed issue, and mandated benefits were repealed at the federal and state levels, health insurance companies could engage in the kind of risk-based underwriting that is taken for granted in other insurance markets. Premiums would be based on expected costs, thereby avoiding adverse selection. Public subsidies could assist those who faced especially high premiums, such as the very sick and elderly, in buying insurance—without any need for a bureaucratically defined minimum-benefits package. Instead of offering a one-size-fits-all plan, firms could compete by offering a variety of insurance products, and individuals and families would have the freedom to buy the kind of health insurance they want.

NOTES

1. Democratic presidential debate sponsored by CNN and the Congressional Black Caucus Institute, January 21, 2008. Retrieved from www.ontheissues.org/2008_cbc_dems.htm.

2. "Obama Flip-flops on Requiring People to Buy Health Care," Politifact.com (*St. Petersburg Times*), www.politifact.com/truth-o-meter/statements/2009/jul/20/barack-obama/obama-flip-flops-requiring-people-buy-health-care/.

3. Robert Moffit, "Obama's Health Reform Isn't Modeled after Heritage Foundation Ideas," *Washington Post*, April 19, 2010. Retrieved from www.washingtonpost.com/wp-dyn/content/article/2010/04/18/AR2010041802727.html. As the article makes clear, Moffit no longer supports the individual mandate. Ronald Bailey, "Mandatory Health Insurance Now!" *Reason Magazine*, November 2004. Retrieved from http://reason.com/archives/2004/11/01/mandatory-health-insurance-now.

4. Economic Report of the President (ERP), February 2010: 186–7.

5. Michael Tanner, "Bad Medicine: A Guide to the Real Costs and Consequences of the New Health Care Law," The Cato Institute (2010):, 5.

6. Ibid.

7. Carla K. Johnson, "Health Premiums Could Rise 17% for Young Adults," Associated Press, March 29, 2010. Retrieved from www.cleveland.com/nation/index.ssf/2010/03/health_premiums_could_rise_17.html.

8. ERP 2010: 203–4.

9. Moffit 2010, for example: "Yes, in the early 1990s, we, along with other prominent conservative economists, supported the idea of such a mandate. It seemed the only way to solve the 'free-rider' problem, in which individuals can, under federal law, walk into any hospital emergency room nationwide and rack up big bills at taxpayer expense."

10. ERP 2010: 187; Hadley, Jack, et al. 2008. "Covering the Uninsured in 2008: Current Costs, Sources of Payment, and Incremental Costs." *Health Affairs*, Web Exclusive 27, no. 5: w399–415.

11. U.S. Department of Health and Human Services, National Health Expenditure Data (Historical), Highlights. Retrieved from www.cms.gov/NationalHealthExpendData/downloads/highlights.pdf.

12. Jack Hadley and John Holohan, "How Much Medical Care Do the Uninsured Use, and Who Pays For It?" *Health Affairs* (February 12, 2003): W3–69 (calculations based on figures in Table 1).

13. Tanner 2010: 8.

14. "Compulsory Auto / Uninsured Motorists," Insurance Information Institute, June 2010. Retrieved from www.iii.org/media/hottopics/insurance/compulsory/.

15. Tanner 2010: 2.

16. The average annual premium for an individual plan in 2009 was $2985. "Individual Health Insurance 2009," AHIP Center for Policy and Research, October 2009: 2. Retrieved from www.ahipresearch.org/pdfs/2009IndividualMarketSurveyFinalReport.pdf.

17. Aaron Yelowitz and Michael F. Cannon, "The Massachusetts Health Plan: Much Pain, Little Gain," The Cato Institute, *Policy Analysis* 657 (January 20, 2010): 3–6. Retrieved from www.cato.org/pubs/pas/pa657.pdf.

18. Kay Lazar, "Short-term Insurance Buyers Drive Up Cost in Mass.," *Boston Globe*, June 30, 2010. Retrieved from www.boston.com/news/health/articles/2010/06/30/short_term_insurance_buyers_drive_up_cost_in_mass/.

19. Michael Tanner, "Massachusetts Miracle or Massachusetts Miserable: What the Failure of the 'Massachusetts Model' Tells Us About Health Care Reform," The Cato Institute, Briefing Paper No. 112, June 9, 2009.

20. Peter Suderman, "Massachusetts Health Program, Model for Obama's Reform, Strains State Budget," *Daily Caller*, January 1, 2010. Retrieved from http://dailycaller.com/2010/01/10/massachusetts-health -program-a-model-for-obamas-national-reform-strains-state-budget/.

21. PPACA, Section 1302(b)(1).

22. PPACA, Section 1302(b)(2).

23. Victoria Craig Bunce and J. P. Wieske, "Health Insurance Mandates in the States 2009," Council for Affordable Health Insurance (2009): 1. Retrieved from www.cahi.org/cahi_contents/resources/pdf/ HealthInsuranceMandates2009.pdf.

24. The number of such mandates increases every year. The equivalent study in 2007 found 1901 mandated benefits, implying that each state passed an average of one more mandated benefit per year. However, some of the new mandates might be newly discovered by the study authors rather than newly passed. Victoria Craig Bunce, J. P. Wieske, and Vlasta Prikazsky, "Health Insurance Mandates in the States 2007," Council for Affordable Health Insurance (2007): 1.

25. Ibid.

26. Amy M. Lischko, "Health Care Premium Expenditures in Massachusetts: Where Does Your Health Care Dollar Go?" Massachusetts Medical Society, undated [c. 2008]. Retrieved from www.massmed .org/AM/Template.cfm?Section=Home6&TEMPLATE=/CM/Content Display.cfm&CONTENTID=22327.

27. Kay Lazar, "Bay State Health Insurance Premiums Highest in Country," *Boston Globe*, August 22, 2009. Retrieved from www.boston .com/news/health/articles/2009/08/22/bay_state_health_insurance _premiums_highest_in_country/.

28. Kevin Sack, "Massachusetts Insurance Regulators Reject Most Requests for Higher Rates," *New York Times*, April 1, 2010. Retrieved from www.nytimes.com/2010/04/02/health/policy/02rates.html.

29. That is, the actuarial value of benefits paid for by the insurance company must equal or exceed 60% of the actuarial value of all benefits. PPACA, Section 1302(c)(1)(A), and Internal Revenue Code of 1986, Section 223(c)(2)(A)(ii).

30. PPACA, Section 1302(d)

3

HEALTH SAVINGS ACCOUNTS AND THE FUTURE OF INSURANCE CHOICE

Grace-Marie Turner

A KEY MOTIVATION for the recent health overhaul law, as stated by President Barack Obama and Congressional leaders, was to increase consumer choice and create a more competitive health insurance market. Ironically, while consumer-directed health plans have been growing in popularity with employers and individual purchasers of health insurance seeking to control rising health costs, the survival of these plans is threatened by the new health overhaul law.

The most popular of the consumer-directed products are Health Savings Accounts (HSAs), enacted by Congress in 2003. The new health overhaul law imposes a number of restrictions on insurance plans that could compromise or even eliminate the HSA option for all but a very few people.

Grace-Marie Turner is president of the Galen Institute, a non-profit research organization focusing on patient-centered health reform initiatives. She can be reached at gracemarie@galen.org.

Ten million Americans now are covered by HSA-qualified health plans, up from eight million last year and six million the year before that, according to the latest survey by America's Health Insurance Plans (AHIP).[1]

People who purchase high-deductible health policies (HDHPs) are allowed to open Health Savings Accounts into which they can deposit money tax-free to pay for health services or save for future needs. These insurance policies generally have lower premiums, and many people and employers use the premium savings to fund the HSAs. The HSA stays with the person as he or she moves from job to job, and the money rolls over from year to year (unlike older Flexible Spending Accounts where you must spend the money by the end of the year or lose it).

Patients like HSAs because they have direct control over their medical spending. That power has yielded relatively low costs as enrollees make their health care dollars work harder. HSAs give consumers a reason to make value-based purchasing decisions, and costs come down. Until now, employers have had the flexibility to tailor benefit and cost structures to fit their budgets and corporate cultures, but the new health overhaul law will limit their options in the future.

Under the new law, the Department of Health and Human Services (HHS) will make the ultimate ruling on HSAs when it decides how to calculate the actuarial value of the high-deductible health insurance policies that must accompany HSAs.

The Patient Protection and Affordable Care Act, signed into law March 23, 2010, requires that all insurance policies provide a minimum actuarial value of at least 60 percent for the benefits covered. If HHS allows contributions by individuals and employers to Health Savings Accounts to "count" as part of the actuarial value, then HSAs and other account-based plans would likely meet the test. But if contributions are not included, the plans likely would not qualify and therefore would not meet the test as a federally-approved insurance product.

In addition, it is uncertain whether high-deductible policies will satisfy the government's legal definition of health insurance that all Americans must carry in order to comply with the federal government's individual mandate, effective 2014. If HHS Secretary Kathleen Sebelius determines that all health plans must include benefits that would violate the HSA guidelines, then HSAs could be effectively outlawed through regulation.

If the health law dooms HSAs, patients would suffer because they would have fewer insurance choices and would be forced to pay for much more extensive and expensive health insurance. Only young adults under age thirty would be able to purchase high-deductible insurance policies and still satisfy the individual mandate for government-approved health insurance.

But even before the regulatory rulings, the overhaul law has claimed the first of what surely will be many victims—a start-up insurance company in Richmond, Virginia, called nHealth. It specialized in insurance plans that coupled HSAs with incentives for wellness, prevention, and assistance in managing chronic illness. Clients loved the innovative health insurance mix that allowed employers and employees to work as partners in getting the best value for their health care dollars.

But the firm's investors saw too many risks ahead to continue to fund the start-up company. "Despite a product that was gaining increasing acceptance among companies throughout the Commonwealth, the uncertainties in the regulatory climate coupled with new demands imposed by national health care reforms have made it challenging to sustain the level of sales required to remain viable over the long run," James Slabaugh, executive vice president of nHealth, said in a letter announcing the company's closing.[2]

nHealth CEO Paul Kitchen said the company was generating revenues and, if allowed to continue, could have turned a profit next year, but investors believed the company's offerings could not comply with all of the new bureaucratic requirements going forward.[3] The company's closure will put fifty employees out of work and denies clients a money-saving health insurance option.

That's unfortunate because most HSA consumers get more value for their health care dollars—an important goal of health reform. When McKinsey and Co., a consulting firm, analyzed the early impact of HSA-compatible health plans nationwide, its researchers found that people with consumer-driven plans were more value conscious.[4] They were 50 percent more likely to ask about costs and three times more likely to choose a less extensive, less expensive treatment option, such as calling a nurse hotline instead of visiting a hospital emergency room. There was no evidence they were skimping on care, and in fact, HSA holders were more likely to get preventive care than those with traditional insurance.

HSA Bank recently released the results of its 2010 Consumer Benchmark Survey, indicating that HSAs have been accepted as a mainstream health coverage option.[5] The data illustrate that people with an HSA-compatible health plan have similar characteristics—including age, health and income—to those with traditional health plans such as HMOs and PPOs:

- 57.5 percent (HSA) and 60.9 percent (traditional) were age 45 or older
- 94.9 percent (HSA) and 93.9 percent (traditional) considered themselves of average or better health
- 44 percent (HSA) and 45 percent (traditional) earned an annual household income ranging from $25,000 to $75,000.

Participation in consumer-directed health plans, as well as health management programs, has been growing over the last few years as companies sought ways to successfully engage employees as partners in managing costs and care. Mercer's latest National Survey of Employer-Sponsored Health Plans found that major employers held total health benefit cost increases per employee to 5.5 percent in 2009— the lowest increase in a decade. (See Figure 3.1 on next page.)[6]

The AHIP study from this year underscores the value of consumer-directed plans in achieving key goals of the health reform effort. Here are some highlights of its survey

FIGURE 3.1
Total health benefit cost increases per employee

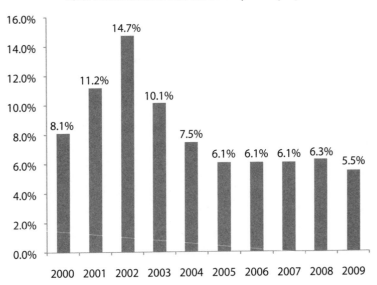

Source: Mercer's National Survey of Employer-Sponsored Health Plans; Bureau of Labor
Statistics, Consumer Price Index, U.S. City Average of Annual Inflation (April to April)
1990–2009; Bureau of Labor Statistics, Seasonally Adjusted Data from the Current
Employment Statistics Survey (April to April) 1990–2009.

showing that 10 million people now are enrolled in HSA-
qualified health insurance:[7]

- *Lower premiums*: Monthly premiums for individuals
  aged 30 to 54 averaged $2,465 a year ($205 a month) and
  $5,335 for a family ($445 a month)—less than half the
  average costs of traditional plans.
- *Larger companies*: The fastest growing market for HSA/
  HDHP products was large-group coverage, which rose by
  one-third, followed by small-group coverage, which grew by
  22 percent.
- *PPOs preferred*: Overall, preferred provider organizations
  (PPOs) were the most popular insurance type, with

88 percent of enrollees. They generally have access to negotiated discount arrangements with health care professionals when paying bills from their HSA accounts.

• More consumer information: More than 90 percent of responding companies reported offering access to HSA account information, health education information, physician-specific information, and personal health records as consumer decision support tools for their members.

• Not just for the young: Fifty-two percent of all individual market enrollees—including dependents covered under family plans—were aged 40 or older so HSAs clearly are not just for the young, as critics claim.

Figures 3.2 and 3.3 tell the story:

FIGURE 3.2
Growth of HSA/HDHP Enrollment from March 2005 to January 2010

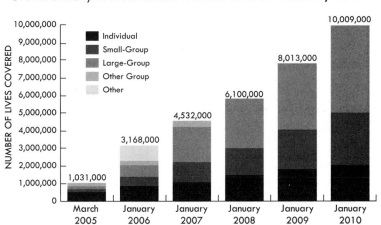

Source: 2010 AHIP HSA/HDHP Census

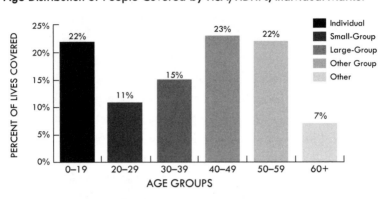

FIGURE 3.3

Age Distribution of People Covered by HSA/HDHPs, Individual Market

Source: 2010 AHIP HSA/HDHP Census

Note: Most enrollers in the 0–19 age group were dependents covered under family plans.

Enrollment in all types of consumer-directed plans over-all grew to an estimated 23 million people in 2009, up from 18 million people in 2008—a 27 percent increase, according to an April report by the American Association of Preferred Provider Organizations.[8]

One example shows why these plans are popular with employees and employers: the state of Utah negotiated an HSA plan to offer to state employees. An article in the *Deseret News* explains that, "Almost any way you look at it, the employee purchasing the HDHP/HSA plan is going to come out ahead":[9]

> For starters, a state employee will pay $685 out of pocket per year in premiums for the traditional family plan. On the other hand, the HDHP/HSA plan is free to the employee.

Once more, the state will be putting $2,340 into a health savings account per year per family (individuals in the state HSA plan receive roughly half of the premium savings and half of the HSA contributions as the families). This means that any employee who opts for the HDHP/HSA plan is already $3,025 ahead of the employee who chooses to stay with the traditional plan. Any employee who spends his or her money wisely and doesn't go over the $2,340 limit gets to keep that money in their HSA for any future health needs, or he or she will be able to withdraw from that account after they retire similar to a 401(k).

If, on the other hand, an employee has an expensive chronic condition or has a catastrophic injury or illness, the HDHP/HSA is still the better way to go. Both the traditional and the HDHP/HSA plan have an out-of-pocket maximum of $7,500, but any money the employee with the HDHP/HSA spends from the HSA will most likely count towards the deductible whereas the $685 that the traditional plan holder spends on premiums does not count. So when both employees reach that $7,500 out-of-pocket maximum, the HDHP/HSA holder has really only spent $5,160, while the traditional plan holder has spent $8,185. Most striking is that the out-of-pocket expenses by the person in the HSA plan can be tax-free while the expenses in the traditional plan are often taxed.

Indiana Governor Mitch Daniels says providing the HSA option to his state's employees will save his state at least $20 million this year, and employees will save $8 million compared to their coworkers in traditional health plans.[10]

More than 70% of Indiana's 30,000 state employees have selected the HSA option.

Governor Daniels says that employees become more active participants in their health care, making smarter and more cost-effective decisions—visiting hospital emergency rooms 67 percent less often and using generic drugs more than those in conventional plans, for example.

Many companies, such as Whole Foods, offer another form of consumer-directed plan called Health Reimbursement Arrangements (HRAs). HRAs give employers more flexibility in shaping their health benefit packages, including the ability to offer account-based plans and provide incentives for prevention and wellness activities. But, unlike HSAs, HRA account balances generally are not portable after employees leave the company.

Both products are helping to make health insurance more affordable and are helping companies to lower health costs.

Washington should make sure that HSAs and other consumer-directed plans remain an option. These plans empower consumers, expand patient choice, and encourage just the sort of responsible medical spending that can drive down health costs.

Competition works when consumers are engaged in getting better value for their health care dollars. nHealth's closing is a warning sign that the new health overhaul law must be stopped before it forces more innovative companies to shut their doors and deprive both individuals and employers of HSAs and other tools they can use to better manage health costs and heath care.

NOTES

1. "January 2010 Census Shows 10 Million People Covered by HSA/ High-Deductible Health Plans," America's Health Insurance Plans, May 2010, at www.ahipresearch.org/pdfs/HSA2010.pdf.

2. Letter from James A. Slabaugh to nHealth agents, June 2, 2010, at www.richmondbizsense.com/images/nhealthletter.pdf.

3. Michael Schwartz, "Startup Health Insurer Shutting," *Richmond BizSense*, June 4, 2010, at www.richmondbizsense.com/2010/06/04/ startup-health-insurer-shutting/.

4. "Consumer-Directed Health Plan Report—Early Evidence Is Promising," McKinsey & Company, June 2005, at http://mckinsey.com/ clientservice/payorprovider/Health_Plan_Report.asp.

5. "2010 Consumer Survey Data Indicates HSAs Are Mainstream Healthcare Option," HSA Bank, June 21, 2010, at http://hsabank.com/ hsabank/General_Info/~/media/Files/Press_Releases/PR062110a.pdf.

6. "In a Tough Year, Employers Hold the Line on Health Benefit Cost Increases," Mercer LLC, November 18, 2009, at www.mercer .com/summary.htm?idContent=1364345.

7. "January 2010 Census Shows 10 Million People Covered by HSA/ High-Deductible Health Plans," America's Health Insurance Plans, May 2010, at www.ahipresearch.org/pdfs/HSA2010.pdf.

8. "Small Employers Lead CDHP Adoption in 2009," American Association of Preferred Provider Organizations (AAPPO), April 14, 2010, at http://aappo.org/UserFiles/File/2010%20CDHP%20Study/ CDHP_Final_web.pdf.

9. Brad Daw, "Health Savings Account the Way to Go for State Employees," *Deseret News*, July 5, 2010, at www.deseretnews.com/ article/700045606/Health-savings-account-the-way-to-go-for-state -employees.html.

10. Governor Mitch Daniels, "Hoosiers and Health Savings Accounts," *The Wall Street Journal*, March 1, 2010, at http://online.wsj .com/article/SB10001424052748704231304575091600470293066.html.

4

MEDICAL INNOVATION IN PERIL

Scott Gottlieb, MD

THE CREATION OF A robust biopharmaceutical and medical device industry is one of modern America's most noteworthy economic and technical achievements. Over the last several decades, advances in diagnostic tests, minimally invasive medical devices, biologics, and small-molecule drugs have improved survival and reduced the physical burdens of a host of maladies. America has led the way in new drug launches and in the development and availability of new devices for safer diagnosis and treatment, to the benefit of patients worldwide. The most visible illustration of these triumphs can be seen in diseases that have benefited from the successive launch of incrementally more effective drugs. Take as an example the treatment of cancer. The overall five-year survival rate for invasive cancers has risen from around 51 percent to almost 70 percent during the last twenty years[1]—the result of better drugs

---

Scott Gottlieb is a resident fellow of the American Enterprise Institute.

being coupled to earlier detection and better treatment protocols. Today, people diagnosed with many early stage cancers cannot only hope for a cure, but should expect one. The overall five-year cancer-free survival rate for early colon cancer is better than 90 percent. Similarly, treatment options for breast cancer have improved overall five-year cancer-free survival to better than 85 percent.[2] Comparable results hold for lymphoma, myeloid leukemia, and other diseases. New medical products aren't the only factor in these gains. But there's no debating that innovative new drugs are having a meaningful impact on these, and many other diseases.

The new health care law specifically targets reimbursement for new drugs and devices as a way to save money in programs like Medicare and Medicaid. These savings, in turn, are used to pay for new health coverage for the uninsured. But the legislation doesn't take down drug and medical device prices directly. Rather, it creates a series of new agencies, boards, and authorities that separately will be empowered to construct new rules to impact how medical products are priced, as well as to restrict their use by defining when and if products are covered by insurance. As this new landscape unfolds over the course of many years, it promises to breed protracted uncertainty about which new medicines or devices will qualify for coverage inside an expanding government-dominated public health sector. These policy steps, and the uncertainty they generate, will inevitably weigh on entrepreneurship, investment, and innovation.

Advocates of these new policies argue that, when it comes to the investments we have made in public and private medical research and in the use of new drugs and medical devices, we aren't getting our money's worth anyway. In this view, a drug development model that isn't working is unlikely to become broken still further by policies that chase away entrepreneurs and investors and otherwise siphon off capital that might have been invested in new endeavors. These critics point to rising investments in research and development set against a flat number of drugs approved by the Food and Drug Administration (FDA) as evidence that more investment is not leading to more breakthroughs. Others assert that no matter how many policies are passed that chip away at the medical products industry, investment in research and development (R&D) will rise because the industry's profits are so vast. Representative Henry Waxman, who has authored many of these policy daggers, has referred to the industry's warnings of declining R&D spending as crocodile tears. He has a chart he brings to the House floor showing that R&D spending continues to rise unabated.

Is this time different? To appreciate, for example, how drug development could be impacted by health reform, one must first accept that better drugs are fueling medical progress. So the case that the innovation model is broken deserves scrutiny. There are many reasons why more research and more drugs entering development haven't led to more drugs being approved. Taken together, they don't reveal an entirely negative story. For one thing, an industry-wide transition from well-understood drug development methods, such as combinatorial chemistry, to more novel platforms has taken drug developers into uncharted areas. This has enabled the development of many effective approaches to targeting disease (the advent of recombinant proteins and monoclonal antibodies as a mainstay of therapies, for example). But it has also led to more dead ends along the way, as uncertainties around new technologies are worked out. Today, a potentially new crop of disruptive modalities is emerging. There is a host of late stage drug candidates predicated on technologies that were largely perfected in just the past ten years. This includes interference RNA (RNAi), therapeutic vaccines, and cell therapy. But all this new science also brings new uncertainties, and a greater chance of failure.

Likewise, new regulatory requirements are also raising the cost of development, prompting companies to shut down even promising development projects as a way to place resources behind the surest bets. By some measures, the average cost of developing a drug has, over the past twenty years, risen at a rate that is 7.4 percent higher than inflation. The same study found that requirements for larger and longer clinical trials were responsible for most of the increase.[3] Another analysis found that total time from synthesis of a new compound to approval averaged 7.9 years in the 1960s, but rose to 12.8 years by the 1990s. Today it is estimated at well over fifteen years. Much of this increased time is spent in the clinical trial phase.[4] (This isn't distributed evenly—drugs for endocrine disorders, for example, spend almost twice as long in clinical testing as antibiotics).[5] These longer development times also mean investments made 10 years ago (such as mapping the human genome, which is expected to increase the number of drug targets by a factor of more than twenty to over

10,000 targets in the near future)[6] are only now showing up in the form of advanced drug candidates and marketed products.[7]

Finally, drug companies are more frequently concluding that the additional cost of continuing development of a drug is not worth its projected returns. In turn, they are voluntarily canceling late stage programs.[8] One older survey of this phenomenon found that between 1981 and 1992, more than 30 percent of curtailed drug programs were shuttered because of "economic reasons".[9] The practice has only grown since. Today, increased competition and more circumspect payers are reducing returns on drugs that aren't sufficiently differentiated from existing compounds. As a result, drug programs are being cancelled in mid stage trials, when the profile of a new medicine starts to more fully emerge. At one time, it would have taken proof that a drug didn't work or that it harbored a safety problem to prompt discontinuation. Now market considerations are leading to the abandonment of drug programs. This is an appropriate market response, but it is nonetheless contributing to fewer new drug launches.

All of these factors have impacted the number of new drugs being approved, making FDA approval statistics a poor proxy for measuring the pace of innovation. The increased novelty of the drugs making it to the market as well as their impact on disease anecdotally tell a much different story. While these features are hard to quantify over the breadth of dozens of product approvals, there's no debating that more of the drugs coming to market are targeted to specific mechanisms of disease, allowing patients to realize more of the benefits and fewer of the side effects of their treatment. An increasing number of drugs are being co-developed with diagnostic tests that enable them to be more precisely targeted to those patients most likely to respond. Moreover, new approaches to drug development—some fashioned in just the last decade such as genomics and proteomics—are already being translated into new medicines. The time between the realization of a basic science principle and its translation into a new therapy is becoming shorter. On the medical device side, advances in microelectronics and materialscience, as well as the increasing coupling of biologics to devices, are leading to a burgeoning of new applications for these products. By all of these measures, and many others, we are in the midst of a biopharmaceutical renaissance.

The question turns to what policy and economic arrangements have enabled this innovation and whether aspects of health reform put these constructs at risk. Steady growth in the capital invested behind research and development is clearly an important factor. Industry participants argue that drug and device industry profits have fueled this investment. There is ample empiric research to support the supposition that profits are reliably recycled into new research and development that in turn fuels additional innovation.[10] But private industry R&D isn't the only capital underpinning research. Others point to the drug industry's typically high profit margins as the differentiating feature. In this scenario, it's the promise of above-average returns on capital that attracts above-average amounts of capital investment and leads to additional research and, in turn, innovation. But taken in the aggregate, returns on invested capital in biotech have been well below other sectors, despite the high profit margins of a small number of highly successful firms. A 2003 analysis of more than 350 publicly traded biotech firms found that only seventy-three produced a positive return on invested capital (ROIC) for the preceding twelve months. Moreover, only half of the firms with a positive ROIC returned more than the weighted average cost of capital (WACC)—a figure used to gauge the opportunity cost of capital.

Given this dismal performance, why do investors fund new biotechs? Entrepreneurs and private investors are chasing the potential to re-price the treatment of a disease with discovery of a major medical improvement and earn significant returns. Much of the private capital for these endeavors is targeted to small biotech companies, which also undertake some of the most creative risk-taking. Because these firms are often dependent on the success of a single product, they embrace more scientific risk than the culture of a big drug company is able to countenance. While the small firms suffer more setbacks as a result, they also produce some of the most significant advances. It is the promise of an outsized return commensurate with the risks and the public health payoff that draws capital to these endeavors. But it is this outsized financial inducement that is put at most risk by elements of health reform. New political constructs make it less likely that public health programs like Medicare will absorb higher prices, even for dramatic improvements in care. Some Wall Street analysts have speculated that a signal of this new government price intolerance may be the Medicare agency's unusually quick action to open a national coverage decision (NCD) when a new prostate cancer therapy called Provenge recently launched at a price that was a premium to existing cancer products.[11] Investors have taken notice. The stock values of leading biotech firms always commanded premium multiples on their earnings. Today, the multiples placed on many top biotech companies (the trading price of their stocks relative to projected earnings) are at near term and in some cases historical lows, reflecting souring investor sentiment for the sector. This limits their ability to raise new capital. Some 75 to 80 percent of biotech companies with market capitalizations under $300 million have valuations that are significantly less than their total capital investment.[12]

The experience of the United Kingdom illustrates the consequence of investor flight from life science ventures. Great Britain has been seen as one of biotech's leading regions. Its 435 public and private biotech companies can claim credit for more than 40% of the biotech products in the pipeline worldwide. Even so, the UK counts few successful commercial ventures among its ranks. Moreover, not a single venture-backed biopharmaceutical product has originated inside a British company.[13] One reason is undercapitalization of these companies—in other words, the absence of private capital to sustain high-risk scientific bets all the way through development. British biotech companies receive on average only 10 to 30 percent of the private investment that is available to their U.S. counterparts.[14] This lack of financing makes it hard to fully develop products, fund expensive development programs, and pay regulatory costs. Ominously, here in the U.S. private capital flows into biotech companies are also declining—a consequence of the economic downturn, but also policy uncertainty that is raising the cost of capital and prompting private investors to flee in favor of other opportunities. Venture capital flows into biotech companies totaled $4.5 billion in 2006, $5.1 billion in 2007, $4.4 billion in 2008 and $3.6 billion in 2009.[15] At the same time, other sectors such as technology and energy have seen relative venture capital flows rise sharply.

Can a British fate await U.S. biotech innovation? If the costs of development continue to increase, and the expected returns are further eroded, then public and private investors are likely to exit the U.S. sector as well. In particular, the ability to "re-price" the treatment of a disease—to command outsized returns to genuine medical advances—is put in doubt as a result of elements of the new health legislation.

Consider first what is meant by the concept of "re-pricing" the treatment of a disease. Take cancer, which accounts for a third of all drugs in development. Cancers that once cost thousands of dollars to treat when there were few effective options now cost tens of thousands with drugs that are dramatically better. One study estimated that the lifetime cost of treating breast cancer in 1984 was, on average, about $37,000. A more recent study of older cancer patients found that just the first twelve months of therapy for earlier-stage breast cancer can top $18,000. Yet the bigger difference isn't the price, but the benefits. Similarly, ten years ago, initial treatment for advanced colon cancer involved a drug regimen that cost hundreds of dollars. Now

initial care that incorporates three new drugs and two biologic drugs costs more than $20,000. But over that time
period, median survival has doubled, and more people with
early stage tumors are using the same drugs to be cured. As
dramatically better treatments came along, the treatment of
these diseases has been "re-priced" higher, but the expected
health benefits have risen exponentially.[16]

This opportunity to earn outsized gains on successful
endeavors is an important aspect of what triggers the capital
investment and risk-taking in drug development. Health
reform will impact this investment model. Indeed, one of
reform's stated goals is to bring closer government scrutiny
to the reimbursement of new medicines. This is being
offered as a way to save money. New government authorities created to scrutinize medical costs will exercise their
mission by capping the upward spiral on drug and medical
device costs. This could diminish the capital formation that
underpins the riskiest endeavors. In particular, health
reform empowers the Centers for Medicare and Medicaid
Services (CMS) to more actively limit coverage and payment. In short time, drug developers will find that they have
to make independent submissions to CMS in order to
secure reimbursement, creating additional uncertainty for
investors. These pricing and coverage decisions will, in turn,
have broad influence across the entire health care market, as
the federal regulation—and the rules hatched by CMS—are
applied to the private health plans sold in the state-based
insurance exchanges that the law creates. The decisions
made by CMS will have a sweeping impact on the choices
available to patients.

Many of the authorities that CMS acquires will flow from the newly created Independent Payment Advisory Board (IPAB), which has the mandate to cut Medicare outlays by $4 billion a year by capping the program's rate of growth. The goal is to keep Medicare's spending growth in line with the overall rate of economic inflation. Since provider groups like hospitals and doctors have gotten themselves exempted from the board's reach, IPAB's focus will fall mostly on drugs and medical devices. The board is also largely barred from setting rules that directly affect access to specific medical products. So IPAB's principal route for reducing Medicare spending is through reductions in what the program pays for individual medical products.

IPAB won't have the time or the clinical capacity to adjudicate the merits of individual medical products. It will instead set broad rules that affect categories of products. IPAB will exercise this capacity through three approaches. First, by taking down the rates that the program pays for products under its existing price schedules. Second, by extending these favorable price schedules to new groups of patients that currently pay market rates (such as expanding the Medicaid best price to the dually eligible patients enrolled in Medicare Part D). Finally, IPAB will achieve its mission by granting CMS authority to more closely adjudicate which technologies the agency will pay for and how it will allow new products to be priced. In other words, it will confer on CMS broad authorities that allow agency staff more discretion in establishing boundaries on coverage, payment, and coding.

It's the latter approach that will have the biggest impact on new investment. IPAB is likely to confer on CMS authority to engage in some tacit forms of reference pricing—fixing reimbursement rates on new products to those paid on similar, but older, and more cheaply priced drugs. One way is by giving CMS the authority to pay only for the "least costly alternative" (LCA) medical product within a broad class of competing treatments. Patients choosing a more costly treatment will have to pay the difference themselves. The Obama administration has already gone to court to fight for this authority prior to the passage of health reform. In that case, a Medicare patient named Ilene Hays sued the federal government after Medicare refused to pay for a medicine a doctor prescribed to treat her obstructive lung disease. The agency only wanted to pay for an older and cheaper substitute. Last year, a court ruled in favor of Hays, arguing that CMS had overstepped its authority. The Obama legal team appealed to the DC Circuit Court and ultimately lost. Now IPAB has the ability to grant this new legal authority to CMS without the need for additional legislation.

That's because IPAB's recommendations won't need a subsequent act of Congress to take full effect. The board's proposals go to Congress, which then has thirty days to either endorse its recommendations, codifying them into law, or come up with a competing proposal that achieves the same degree of Medicare savings. In this way, the board's charter is designed to leverage Congress' inability to act in a timely fashion. It is highly unlikely that Congress can draft, propose, and pass any legislative scheme in thirty days, not to mention one as politically contentious as a plan

for cutting Medicare spending. As a result, the IPAB proposals are likely to take effect by virtue of Congressional
inaction. IPAB was designed with this goal in mind.
IPAB is also likely to give CMS broad authority to establish new linkages between the CMS coding and coverage
processes. This is another administrative tool for referenc-
ing the prices of new products to older alternatives. By
giving new products the same code as cheaper alternatives,
Medicare can pay a category of products the same rate
even if a newer alternative is differentiated in a way that
gives it added advantages to patients. Medicare wants to
be able to exert this leverage to compel product developers
to file submissions with the agency (presumably supported
by unique clinical studies) whenever a sponsor wants to
achieve premium reimbursement over a current standard
of care.

While proponents of IPAB will argue that its process will
recognize innovation and reward it appropriately, there is
little to suggest this will be the case. On the contrary, when
CMS has been given discretion to set coverage policies and
payment rates, it has often been preoccupied with cost over
clinical benefit. Take the agency's tortured decisions around
the use of implantable defibrillators that shock stopped
hearts to prevent sudden death. Medicare sharply restricted
use of them 1990s. But mounting research proved that the
devices, which cost $30,000, could be saving many more
lives. So in 2003 Medicare adopted a novel theory to expand
coverage to some, but not everyone who needed one. The
agency said that only patients with certain measures on

their electrocardiograms (called wide QRS) seemed to benefit.[17] It was an easily measurable but ultimately imprecise way to allocate the devices. After another major study firmly debunked the QRS theory, Medicare expanded coverage again in 2005, potentially saving 2,500 additional lives, according to its press release issued with that decision.[18] That experience wasn't unique. From 1999 to 2007 Medicare denied access to a third of the treatments it evaluated through its coverage process, taking an average of eight months to complete reviews. When coverage was granted, in 85 percent of cases the treatments were restricted, usually to patients with more advanced illnesses.[19]

The problem is that this CMS process is likely to remain unpredictable, opaque, and poorly informed for many years. Processes for decision making inside CMS have historically been ad hoc. This is especially true relative to its sister agency, FDA, which has established predictable procedures for how it evaluates products and reaches its decisions. CMS has far fewer formal procedures and public disclosure governing its coverage and payment process. The agency's staff has historically been resistant to efforts aimed at getting it to define in guidance or regulation the criteria they use to reach decisions. CMS has also been plagued by difficulty attracting and retaining qualified personnel. To give one proxy, CMS has fewer than twenty physicians on its coverage staff and fewer than forty total clinicians once pharmacists, nurses, and other health care providers are counted. While this isn't a precise surrogate for sound decision-making, it gives insight into how well the agency informs its decisions. Most of its physicians are generalists.

It doesn't have a single oncologist on its staff, and has just one nephrologist despite the fact that it pays for the vast majority of dialysis performed in the U.S. To give a basis for comparison, private health plans—which exercise far fewer authorities to set prices or coverage rules—have more clinicians by order of magnitude on their staffs. Aetna has more than 140 physicians and about 3,300 nurses, pharmacists and other clinicians. Wellpoint has 4,000 clinicians across its different businesses, including 125 doctors and 3,180 nurses. United Healthcare employs about 600 doctors and 12,000 clinicians across its health care businesses.[20]

Higher reimbursement uncertainty is already chasing investment capital into other endeavors that are more lucrative when adjusted for their risk. Venture capital funds are shifting new resources into more favored technology spaces such as clean energy. Big pharmaceutical companies are diversifying into animal health, generics, and cosmetics.

Capital will flow to the areas of highest risk-adjusted returns. There's no reason drug companies need to stay in the business of developing ethical drugs. Device companies can similarly diversify away from surgical products. We have seen drug companies diversify away from medical research before as a response to periods of political and policy uncertainty. Drug companies will also focus much more attention and resources on maximizing sales of existing products. Investments in marketing current drugs may increase relative to investments in R&D. They will also see consolidation as a key strategy for gaining leverage to counter the greater power of the government buyers. The net result will be that the industry's total R&D effort is going to shrink. Instead of thirty or so medium-to-large companies we will have perhaps a dozen behemoths spending half or one-quarter of the same amount.[21]

New authorities such as IPAB will increase uncertainty around how products will be reimbursed, ultimately discouraging investment and risk-taking. The ensuing policy limbo is likely to persist for decades as agencies work out how they will exercise their new tools. Investors will shun the field, and scientific risk-taking will diminish. As experience in the UK biotech sector shows, once capital flees the life sciences in favor of other endeavors, it does not necessarily return.

NOTES

1. Surveillance, Epidemiology, and End Results (SEER) Program 2010, National Cancer Institute.

2. Abenaa M. Brewster, et al, "Residual Risk of Breast Cancer Recurrence 5 Years After Adjuvant Therapy." *Journal of the National Cancer Institute* 100 (2008): 1179–1183.

3. C. Johnston, *Annals of Neurology* 62[6] (2007): A6–7.

4. J. A. DiMasi, R. W. Hansen, and H. G. Gradbowski, "The Price of Innovation: New Estimates of Drug Development Costs," *Journal of Health Economics* 22 (2003)151–185.

5. Editorial, "The Numbers Game," *Nature Drug Discovery* 1 (2002): 929.

6. Oliver Gassmann, Gerrit Reepmeyer, and Maximilian von Zedtwitx, "The Science and Technology Challenge: How to Find New Drugs," *Leading Pharmaceutical Innovation.* Berlin & Heidelberg: Springer, 2008), 33–49.

7. S. Gottlieb, "Two Steps Forward in the War against Cancer." *Wall Street Journal,* June 9, 2010, A24.

8. M. Dickson and J. P. Gagnon, "Key Factors in the Rising Cost of New Drug Discovery and Development," *Nature Reviews* 3 (2004): 417–429.

9. J. DiMasi, "Risks in New Drug Development: Approval Success Rates for Investigational Drugs," *Clinical Pharmacology & Therapeutics* (May 2001): 297–307.

10. U. E. Reinhardt, "Perspectives On The Pharmaceutical Industry: Granting all Americans Access to Prescription Drugs that Work Should Be a Trivial Economic Challenge for This Wealthy Nation," *Health Affairs* 5 (2001): 136–149; C. Giaccotto, R. Santerre, J. Vernon, "Explaining Pharmaceutical R&D Growth Rates at the Industry Level: New Perspectives and Insights," AEI-Brookings Joint Center for Regulatory Studies, White Paper (2003); H. Grabowski and J. Vernon, "The Determinants of Pharmaceutical Research and Development Expenditures," *Journal of Evolutionary Economics* 10 (2000): 201–215; T. A. Abbotta and J. Vernon, "The Cost of US Pharmaceutical Price Regulation: A Financial Simulation Model of R&D Decisions," *Managerial and Decision Economics* 28 (2007): 293–306.

11. "Provenge NCA Likely to Support On-Label Coverage Inquiry Not Part of Wider Attack on Biologic Coverage, The Marwood Group Report, July 6, 2010.

12. May 2010 health care private equity roundtable discussion sponsored by Morgan Stanley, a transcript of which was published in Morgan Stanley's *Journal of Applied Corporate Finance.*

13. G. Smith, S. M. Akram, K. Redpath, and W. Bains, "Wasting Cash—the Decline of the British Biotech Sector, *Nature Biotechnology* 6 (2009): 531–537.

14. P. Mitchell, *Nature Biotechnology* 23 (2005):1029.

15. PricewaterhouseCoopers/National Venture Capital Association MoneyTreeTM Report, Data: Thomson Reuters Total U.S. Investments by Year Q1 1995—Q2 2010, July 16, 2010; D. C. Ackerly, A. M.Valverde, L. W. Diener, K. L. Dossary, K. A. Schulman, "Fueling Innovation In Medical Devices (And Beyond): Venture Capital In Health Care," *Health Affairs* 28 (January/February 2009): w68–w75.

16. S. Gottlieb, "How Obama Would Stifle Drug Innovation," *Wall Street Journal,* October 18, 2008, A22.

17. M. B. McClellan and S. R. Tunis, "Medicare Coverage of ICDs," *New England Journal of Medicine* 352 (2005): 222–224.

18. CMS Press Release, "Medicare Expands Coverage of Implantable Defibrillators to Save Lives and Develop Evidence to Maximize Benefits," January 27, 2005, available at www.cms.hhs.gov/apps/media/press/release.asp?counter=1331

19. P. J. Neumann, M. S. Kamae, J. A. Palmer, "Medicare's National Coverage Decisions For Technologies, 1999–2007," *Health Affairs* 6 (2008): 1620–1631.

20. S. Gottlieb, "What's at Stake in the Medicare Showdown," *Wall Street Journal*, June 24, 2008.

21. "The Campaign Against Innovation," Speech by Sidney Taurel, president, chief executive officer, delivered at the American Enterprise Institute, Washington, DC, March 18, 2003.

5

THE REAL MATH OF CONGRESSIONAL BUDGET OFFICE ESTIMATES

Douglas Holtz-Eakin

THE UNITED STATES faces a daunting budgetary outlook, with the administration's budget displaying an unsustainable debt spiral emerging over the next decade. In this context, the fiscal consequences of the newly enacted Patient Protection and Affordable Care Act (PPACA) are central to any evaluation of its desirability.

Advocates for the act defend its budgetary integrity by pointing to the Congressional Budget Office (CBO) "score" that suggests a modest contribution to deficit reduction over the budget window and beyond. Alternatively they argue that the CBO understates the beneficial impacts of the Act on the pace of health care spending.

This strikes me as wishful thinking, at best. As outlined below, the budgetary framework for the act relies on budget

Douglas Holtz-Eakin is the president of the American Action Forum. The opinions expressed herein are those of the author and not the American Action Forum.

gimmicks, politically unrealistic spending reductions and tax increases that will fail to offset the introduction of new entitlement spending. As a result, the act will serve to accelerate the coming fiscal crisis.

THE APPROACHING FISCAL TRAIN WRECK

The unsustainable nature of the federal budget over the long term has been outlined in successive versions of the CBO's Long-Term Budget Outlook. In broad terms, over the next thirty years, the inexorable dynamics of current law will raise outlays, or committed federal expenditures, from about 20 percent of gross domestic product (GDP) to anywhere from 30 to 40 percent of GDP.[1] If policy makers attempt to keep taxes at their postwar norm of 18 percent of GDP, the result will be an unmanageable federal debt spiral. In contrast, a strategy of ratcheting up taxes to match spending appetite would likely be self-defeating as it would undercut badly needed economic growth.

Setting aside how one measures the size of the problem, its character is clear: spending rises above any reasonable level of tax receipts for the indefinite future. Accordingly, over the long term, the budget problem is primarily a spending problem and correcting it requires reductions in the growth of large mandatory spending programs and the appetite for federal outlays.

The most recent Administration budget shows that the long-standing problem has become dramatically worse and a crisis will arrive more quickly. The federal government ran a fiscal 2009 deficit of $1.4 trillion—the highest since World War II—as spending reached nearly 25 percent of GDP and receipts fell below 15 percent of GDP. In each case, the levels are unlike those experienced during the last fifty years.

Going forward, there is no relief in sight. Over the next ten years, according to the CBO's analysis of the President's Budgetary Proposals for fiscal year 2011, the deficit will never fall below $700 billion dollars.[2] In 2020, the deficit will be 5.6 percent of GDP, roughly $1.3 trillion, of which over $900 billion will be devoted to servicing debt on previous borrowing.

The budget outlook is not the result of a shortfall of revenues. The CBO projects that over the next decade the economy will fully recover and revenues in 2020 will be 19.6 percent of GDP—over $300 billion more than the postwar average of 18 percent of GDP. Instead, the problem is spending. Federal outlays in 2020 are expected to be 25.2 percent of GDP—about $1.2 trillion higher than the 20 percent that has been usual in the postwar era.

As a result of the spending binge, in 2020 public debt will have more than doubled from its 2008 level to 90 percent of GDP and will continue its upward trajectory. The treacherous budgetary waters facing the United States make close scrutiny of the act not only appropriate, but essential.

THE PATIENT PROTECTION AND
AFFORDABLE CARE ACT

The final score of the Patient Protection and Affordable Care Act with reconciliation amendments was released publicly on March 20, 2010.[3] The CBO and Joint Committee on Taxation estimated the act would lead to a net reduction in federal deficits of $143 billion over ten years with $124 billion in net reductions from health care reform and $19 billion derived from education provisions. (I ignore the latter in what follows.)

This bottom line shows the net effect of multiple spending and receipts provisions. Total subsidies in the act exceed $1 trillion dollars over ten years and include insurance exchange tax credits for individuals, small employers tax credits, the creation of reinsurance and high risk pools, as well as expansions to Medicaid and the Children's Health Insurance Program. To finance the subsidies and reduce the deficit, total cost savings are projected to be nearly $500 billion based on reductions in annual updates to Medicare fee-for-service payment rates, Medicare Advantage rates, and Medicare and Medicaid disproportionate share hospital (DSH) payments. In addition to the cost-saving measures, the act raises more than $700 billion in tax revenue from reinsurance and risk adjustment collections, penalty payments by employers and uninsured individuals, an excise tax on high-premium plans, fees on manufacturers and insurers, and other revenue provisions.

To gain a rough feel of the longer-run impacts, I extrapolated the budgetary impacts for the years 2020 to 2029 using

CBO's estimated compounded annual growth rates. Under this crude approach, the act is expected to yield an additional $681 billion in deficit reduction.

Taken at face value, then, the act provides both near-term and longer-run budgetary savings. This is quite a striking finding in light of the fact that the act sets up two new entitlement spending programs (insurance subsidies and long-term care insurance), each of which is projected to grow indefinitely at an annual rate of 8 percent for the foreseeable future. Can the assertion of budgetary savings really be true? The answer, unfortunately, appears to be no.

A more realistic assessment emerges if one strips out gimmicks and budgetary games and reworks the calculus. Doing so suggests a very different picture: the act would raise, not lower, federal deficits, by $554 billion in the first ten years and $1.4 trillion over the succeeding ten years.[4]

The first step in reworking the calculus is to note that substantial costs are simply omitted from the CBO score. To operate the new health care programs over the first ten years, future Congresses will need to vote for $274.6 billion in additional spending in the next ten years. This unbudgeted spending includes the discretionary costs for the Internal Revenue Service (IRS) to enforce and the Centers for Medicare and Medicaid Services (CMS) to administer insurance coverage, explicitly authorized health care grant programs, and the Medicare Physician Payment Reform Act, which revises the sustainable growth rate for physician reimbursement. All of these provisions are noted in CBO's report but none of them is factored into the final score of the act.

The next adjustment centers on spending cuts that ultimately the CMS will likely be unable to implement. These are composed of cost reductions through Medicare market basket updates, the Independent Payment Advisory Board, Medicare Advantage interactions, and the Part D premium subsidy for high-income beneficiaries. While the specifics of each differ, these provisions share two features. First, the act does not fundamentally reform Medicare in such a manner that will permit it to operate at lower budgetary cost. Accordingly, when the time comes to implement these savings (or those developed by the Independent Payment Advisory Board) CMS will be faced with the possibility of strongly limited benefits, the inability to serve beneficiaries, or both. As a result, the cuts will be politically infeasible, as Congress is likely to continue to regularly override scheduled cuts.

Second, it is reasonable to question the political willingness of Congress to actually impose the excise tax on high-premium, "Cadillac," health plans. This tax was supposed to start immediately according to the Senate's version of the Patient Protection and Affordable Care Act. After intense lobbying by organized labor, Congress relented and pushed the tax back to 2018. This raises the possibility that it will prove politically infeasible to ever implement the tax. (Indeed, this has been the experience of politically unpopular cuts imposed on physician reimbursement by the sustainable growth rate formula—they are not permitted to occur.) If so, there will be a loss of $78 billion in revenues over the next ten years.

The final gimmick is to double-count premiums for the CLASS Act (premiums for long-term care insurance) and the potential increase in Social Security receipts. In principal, these receipts should be reserved to cover future payments and not be devoted to short-term deficit reduction. The CLASS Act premiums total $70 billion over the first ten years, while the PPACA also uses $53 billion for deficit reduction from an anticipated increase in Social Security tax revenue. The CBO estimates that outlays for Social Security benefits would increase by only about $2 billion over the 2019 period, and that the coverage provisions would have a negligible effect on the outlays for other federal programs. If Social Security revenues do rise as employers shift from paying for health insurance to paying higher wages, the extra money raised from payroll taxes should be preserved for the Social Security trust fund.

As noted above, incorporating all of these adjustments yields a radically different bottom line. The act generates additional deficits of $562 billion in the first ten years. And, as the nation would be on the hook for two more entitlement programs rapidly expanding as far into the future as we can envision, the deficit in the second ten years would approach $1.5 trillion.

If this were not sobering enough, there is the real risk that the insurance subsidies will be substantially more expensive than anticipated. For better or (more likely) worse, health insurance is heavily entangled with the labor market. Today about 163 million workers and their families receive health insurance coverage from their employers and about one-half of the act's spending is for insurance subsidies. The subsidies are remarkably generous, even for those with relatively high incomes. For example, a family earning about $59,000 a year in 2014 would receive a premium subsidy of about $7,200. A family making $71,000 would receive about $5,200, and even a family earning about $95,000 would receive a subsidy of almost $3,000.

These subsidies threaten to induce a large number of employers to drop their insurance plans, with the complete concurrence of their employees. Thus, the key question is whether the employer can keep the employee "happy"— appropriately compensated and insured—and save money.

The answer is frequently "yes"—thanks to the generosity of federal subsidies.[5] For example, for a worker with an income of $59,250 (250 percent of the Federal Poverty Level) the employer could drop $12,000 in insurance, pay the $2,000 penalty the PPACA imposes on doing so, give the worker a raise of $8,391 and pocket a tidy $1,550. Importantly, the worker could use her raise and the $7,530 subsidy to purchase insurance as good as what she gave up. What's not to like—as long as taxpayers are financing the deal?

The potential impact is quite large. At present there are 123 million Americans at or below this income cutoff. Roughly 60 percent of Americans work; about 60 percent of those receive employer-sponsored insurance. A conservative estimate suggests that there could be 35 to 40 million workers who might receive subsidies. In contrast, CBO estimated that only 19 million residents would receive subsidies, at a cost of about $450 billion over the first 10 years. This analysis suggests that the number could as much as triple (19 million plus an additional 38 million in 2014) meaning that the gross price tag would be $1.4 trillion.

CONCLUSION

The budgetary stakes could not be higher. Unfortunately, the putative deficit reduction from the act is built on a shaky foundation of omitted costs, premiums shifted from other entitlements, and politically dubious spending cuts and revenue increases. And the underlying entitlement may prove to be much more expensive than anticipated.

The future of the Patient Protection and Affordable Care Act is likely even more important than its passage. In light of the extraordinarily precarious state of federal fiscal affairs and the enormous downside risks presented by the act, one can only hope that every future effort is devoted to reducing its budgetary footprint.

NOTES

1. Congressional Budget Office, *The Long-Term Budget Outlook*. Washington, DC: Congress of the United States; 2009 June.

2. Congressional Budget Office, *An Analysis of the President's Budgetary Proposals for Fiscal Year 2011*. Washington, DC: Congress of the United States; 2010 March.

3. Congressional Budget Office. H.R. 4872, Reconciliation Act of 2010. Washington, DC: Congress of the United States; 2010 March.

4. See Douglas Holtz-Eakin and Michael J. Ramlet, "Health Care Reform Is Likely To Widen Federal Budget Deficits, Not Reduce Them" *Health Affairs* 29, no. 6 (2010): 1136–1141.

5. See Douglas Holtz-Eakin and Cameron Smith,"Labor Markets and Health Care Reform: New Results," http://americanactionforum .org/files/LaborMktsHCRAAF5-27-10_0.pdf

6

THE IMPERFECT ART OF MEDICAL MALPRACTICE REFORM

Richard A. Epstein

T HE GREATEST TRANSFORMATION of the health care delivery system in the United States was put in place in March 2010 when President Barack Obama and a Democratic congress prevailed over a fierce but unavailing Republican opposition. The Patient Protection and Affordable Care Act[1]—aka ObamaCare—alters, in unimagined ways, the tax and regulatory environment for the delivery of health care services in the public and private spheres. Yet in the midst of all that tumult, Congress pointedly chose to bypass one area of passionate interest to doctors, hospitals, and other health care providers: the much

Richard A. Epstein is the Peter and Kirsten Bedford Senior Fellow at the Hoover Institution. He is the Laurence A. Tisch Professor of Law at New York University and the James Parker Hall Distinguished Service Professor of Law at the University of Chicago. My thanks to Brett Davenport, Maxine Sharavsky, and Christopher Tan, NYU Law School, Class of 2012, for their valuable research assistance.

mooted issue of medical malpractice reform. ObamaCare's unmemorable contribution to this arena was its "sense of the Senate" (but not of the House of Representatives) in support of some modest experimental projects at the state level, which at some far distant time might disclose some undefined improvements within the system.

The realist explanation for the want of any meaningful medical malpractice reform starts and ends with the proposition that the Democratic Party is joined at the hip to one of its key constituent groups: the trial lawyers. The more charitable explanation is that medical malpractice reform does not exert sufficient influence on the overall operation of the health care system to merit that inclusion in major social legislation. There is obvious truth in the former proposition, but much controversy over the latter. The substantive question is: Just what could any Congress hope to achieve by intelligent medical malpractice reform? Answering that question is not easy. It is first necessary to grasp the situation on the ground with medical malpractice. Just how many resources does it consume, and what social dislocations, if any, does it create? Once that is done, it is possible to think about a range of reforms and their probable consequences. Part I of this paper thus gives a brief overview of costs, direct and indirect, of running the current liability system. Part II then turns to a theoretical discussion of the proper basis of medical malpractice liability in order to explain why private contracts, not public tort rules, should govern. Part III then examines the set of possible reforms that could respond to the theoretical difficulties in the current approach. A brief conclusion follows.

MACRO AND MICROTRENDS
IN MEDICAL MALPRACTICE

Just what does medical malpractice do to the cost and quality of health care? The analysis of this question starts with a simple pair of questions. First, what is the direct cost of medical malpractice in the United States? Second, what are the indirect costs from defensive medicine? On the first of these questions, the estimates of direct medical malpractice outlays are indeed too small to drive the overall costs of the health care system. The usual estimates place that figure at well under 1 percent of the overall total of health care costs, and usually around half that number.[2] In real terms, these health care costs usually increase more in a year than the total costs of running the malpractice system. Judged by this standard, the entire direct payout with respect to medical malpractice looks and feels like a rounding error. The percentage of the gross domestic product (GDP) devoted to health care expenditures in 1960 was about 5.2 percent. It reached 17.3 percent in 2009, with annual increases of about 6.7 percent[3]—real money, but those sums are not large enough to make a decisive difference in the operation of the overall health care system, which consumes many multiples of these sums on a routine basis. Direct medical malpractice may strike with special fury on certain specialties in certain locales, but in terms of overall costs, the number is small.

The great unknown in this area, however, is the extent of "defensive medicine," which includes all those extra expenditures that are made not to deal with patient well-being, but to insulate physicians from potential liability for adverse outcomes. Those estimates vary widely, but are said in some instances to equal around 10 percent of overall health care expenditures, which would put it at an implausible $250 billion per year. A recent survey in the Archives of Internal Medicine relied on survey data to establish a figure less than a quarter of that amount at $60 billion, or, in other words, slightly above 2 percent of total system costs.[4] The United States Department of Health and Human Services estimates the range at between $70–$126 billion; a Stanford research team puts the range at between $84–$151 billion, and National Center for Policy Research has it somewhat lower at $50–$110 billion.[5] Using a figure of $100 billion dollars translates into about a 4 percent rate of expenditure for defensive medicine out of the roughly $2.5 trillion that the United States spends on health care.[6] The AMA study also estimated that the direct costs of running the malpractice system totaled about 2 percent of the total outlay, or 5 percent.

The estimates of direct expenditures are relatively accurate. Those for defensive medicine are, at best, an educated guess, given the huge difficulties in isolating and costing out these expenditures. Thus, on the one hand, many of these defensive procedures may well provide some improvement, but not at the level that would be regarded as cost-justified. On the other hand, the extra test that is not cost-justified need not be completely wasteful either, even when compared to the next best course of action. Pricing that component of defensive medicine is thus difficult. Do we include the entire expenditure in the defensive medicine category, or only the excess? There is a huge diversity of procedures in a wide range of institutional settings. Making the proper allocations is a fool's errand, even for experts armed with the most sophisticated econometric techniques. The number is surely positive, probably large, but ultimately elusive. I have just given one set of reasons why those estimates of defensive medicine may be too high. It is also possible to identify areas in which the estimates are too low. Medical malpractice is a cost of doing business. One of its hidden costs could well stem from the unwillingness of physicians and hospitals to enter into various kinds of transactions at all. In some cases, the breakdown is slow. Obstetricians stop delivering babies or retire early. Neurosurgeons leave one state to set up shop across the border. In other instances, it can be more dramatic, with insistent legislative protests.

Again, it is difficult to measure the full extent of these losses. But on balance, I think that it is fair to say that the confident thesis that medical malpractice liability is the driver of increased costs is surely overstated. But suppose it is small, relative to the enormous costs of the health care system. What follows from this proposition? Perhaps it need not be the centerpiece of a national debate on health care that is dominated by the traditional triad of access, cost, and quality of care. But with that debate over, surely a $25 or $50 billion problem is worth some serious study when no one thinks that the status quo gets us as a nation close to the right solution.

On this point, we do not have to look to sophisticated econometric evidence. The behavioral evidence of physicians and hospitals confirms that something is amiss. In successful markets, firms do not constantly threaten to reduce their operations or close up shop altogether. Indeed, in the health care setting, if medical malpractice liability produced benefits in excess of the associated costs, who would object? No longer would malpractice liability function as a drag on the system. The private right to sue badly behaving physicians would be treated as a welcome deterrent. The improved performance of the system would make this liability tax well worth paying. Patients who might otherwise be on the fence could have the additional assurance needed to seek risky medical treatment or complex procedures, knowing that the increase in fees is more than offset by the reduction in risk.

Yet this scenario never plays out. Without question, all the private adaptations to higher liability have reduced the range of available services. Obstetricians stopped delivering babies out of fear of medical malpractice liability. Texas was losing physicians until an aggressive 2003 reform of medical malpractice liability capped noneconomic damages at $250,000, thereby inducing a sharp influx of physicians in response to the favorable liability environment. The liability cap also led to a decrease in insurance premiums, by around 27 percent. The change in the law also increases the odds that the favorable environment will last for longer periods of time, which allows physicians to make their front-end investments within the state, confident that they will be able to reap a return in future years. These inflows work to advance consumer welfare by affording greater access to health care. Successful treatments provide huge personal gains in the form of longer life spans and lower levels of pain and disability.

At the ground level, the serious flaws of the medical malpractice system seem evident. Its administrative costs are high, but its deterrent effects are at best modest. Here are some pointers in that direction. A 2006 study in the *New England Journal of Medicine* concluded that the administrative expenses of the malpractice system were "exorbitant."[7] Worse, the study found errors in jury verdicts in about one-quarter of the litigated cases. Juries denied compensation properly due in 16 percent of the cases, and awarded it about 10 percent of the time when it was unwarranted. These error calculations don't include damage awards set at improper levels. Unfortunately, these high error rates effectively undercut the deterrence effect of the system, leaving open the prospect that other forms of oversight—by hospital review boards, for example—might provide prompter, cheaper, and more reliable forms of oversight.

Some comparative evidence reinforces the claim that the American malpractice system is overheated. As a general matter, no other nation has a level of malpractice that rivals the size and complexity of ours. Yet there is little evidence that the higher level of liability generates higher levels of care. A careful Canadian study from the early 1990s, carried out by Donald Dewees and Michael Trebilcock, concluded that the Canadian levels of medical malpractice were about the same as U.S. levels—for about 10 percent of the total cost.[8] One can argue about the extent of the disarray, but not about the fact of disarray. To understand how this comes to pass, it is necessary to examine the theoretical foundations for medical malpractice liability.

MEDICAL MALPRACTICE—
TORT OR CONTRACT?

The persistent disruptions and disputes over medical malpractice are stark evidence of the basic flaw in the design of the system. The best way in which to understand this point is to back off the innocent but misleading description of medical malpractice as an issue that requires tort reform. The prior question asks, why treat medical malpractice as a regime of tort law in the first place? Under common understanding today, a tort case arises whenever there is bodily injury or property damage. Only the former is at stake in medical malpractice. The usual implication of calling something a tort means that positive law fixes the rights and duties of the parties as a matter of public policy. That approach is surely inescapable in cases involving strangers where the harm is inflicted on some person with whom the actor has no antecedent relationship. In these cases, the only expectation that any person has of a stranger is that he keep his hands to himself. If he does not, he should ideally pay damages that put the injured party back in his previous position, to the extent that money can accomplish this.

With health care services, the patient does not want a doctor or nurse to act like a stranger, taking care only to avoid contact. She wants that person to take care of her, i.e., expend attention, labor, and resources on her. Those all cost money, and the system will only remain viable if the revenues received by caregivers—net other expenses of running the system—are sufficient to cover all liability awards, plus the costs of defending all suits, meritorious or not, while allowing for a reasonable rate of return on invested capital. At this point, a damage rule that pays all damages in full is plainly unsustainable. The surgeon cannot be responsible for the physical dislocations from every incision; the physician cannot be responsible for all the adverse side effects of medicines. It is the nature of medical care that efforts that have only a chance of improving health also have a certainty of inflicting some known and well-understood harm. If the compensate-all-losses regime dominated, no one could afford to supply medical services because their customers would not be able to afford the lavish coverage of compensating future losses from health care treatments that, on average, have been to the benefit of the patient.

Here are some numbers to illustrate the dangers of over-extensive liability. Suppose a surgery has a 50 percent chance to succeed, which on success produces $100,000 in benefits. Suppose, too, that in 1 percent of the cases, the outcome will be worse than the original condition, yielding a $500,000 loss. In the other 49 percent of the cases, there are no changes. The expected gain from this operation is $50,000 ($0.5 \times \$100,000 = \$50,000$) less the $5,000 (or $500,000 \times 0.01$) cost of an adverse event. The net expected value of the surgery is $45,000 to the plus side, which most informed people will eagerly accept. But if, after the fact, liability is owing in the 1 percent of bad outcome cases, it adds $5,000 to the bill, plus an allowance for litigation fees. In costly medical malpractice cases, these costs are, on average for both sides, easily equal to the expected losses, or, say, another $5,000. To use the regime of automatic compensation for all harms adds on to these numbers $10,000 to the cost of providing services. That is money that most people don't have for a procedure that might otherwise cost only $2,000. This strict liability for all losses shuts down services that the patient desperately wants to have.

No one wants that result, and the question is how best to cut back from it. The usual first answer is to leave the measure of damages constant, but to cut down on the frequency of liability so that the full $500,000 becomes payable in fewer cases. Liability is thus restricted to cases of negligence. Compensation is only payable if the physician deviated from the standard of care followed by physicians in his line of practice. Suppose that negligence rule were to knock out liability 90 percent of the time. On the numbers above, the expected liability costs of treatment go down from $5,000 to $500. The anticipated litigation expenses go down the same amount. The narrower base of liability thus adds only $500 on a $2,000 procedure, a number that is noticeable but not insuperable.

These are just illustrative numbers. Whether the negligence standard works to slim down liability depends on the real numbers. Before, roughly speaking, 1960, the law of medical malpractice was tilted toward defendants, who got the benefit of the doubt on virtually every aspect of the case. The standard of care was formally negligence, but the deference toward physicians drove that negligence standard away from the tougher liability rules used in stranger cases to a softer rule that required a plaintiff, in practice, to show something closer to gross negligence—or a systematic disregard of customary standard—to win on liability. In addition, the other key elements of proof, dealing with causation and damages, were also resolved favorably to defendants. In aggregate, the total costs of running that earlier malpractice system were so low that no physician or hospital, thought it worthwhile to contract away from these liability rules. To use our numbers empirically, the add-on for liability for the $2,000 procedure would not be $500, but $5. Not a big deal.

In the late 1950s, however, the foundations of the older liability system began to receive popular and academic scrutiny. The older attitudes of deference toward doctors and hospitals started to give way. A new era of judicial and popular suspicion toward health care providers grew in its place. Hospitals and physicians began to ask for various waivers as a condition for supplying treatment. But it did not work. Court after court decided that these waivers should be regarded as invalid,[9] or that they should be read narrowly in favor of patients.[10] It was not just one single change that made the liability system seem untenable. It was the synergistic effect of multiple small changes in the legal rules and jury attitudes on such topics as expert witnesses, informed consent, the standard of care, proof, causation, and, especially, damages, that altered the basic equation.

The doctrinal changes the practice landscape. By the early to mid-1970s, both the frequency and severity of potential liability pushed that liability higher in select areas, to the point that promising but risky medical procedures carried high medical malpractice price tags. The ebbs and flows in the last thirty-five years have not restored matters to the pre-1960 equilibrium. To be sure, the increased rates of insurance can reflect, in part, the bad performance of investment portfolios. But just because the stock market performs poorly does not automatically mean that premiums should be higher. After all, doctors and groups that self-insured would also have to put aside larger sums to meet their self-insured liabilities. That said, the change in investment conditions does not eliminate the role that the steady expansion of medical malpractice liability had in the post-1960 period. So the practical task now becomes simple: What can be done to shrink the malpractice liability so that the anticipated gains from sensible health care treatment can be realized? It is this point we can turn to as the possible reform approaches.

THE IMPERFECT ART OF MEDICAL MALPRACTICE REFORM

There are two—and only two—possible ways to reduce the frequency and severity of the liability payments derived from providing health care. The first is contractual and the second is statutory.

Contractual fixes

The first and most radical approach, which I have advocated now for close to thirty-five years,[11] is to replace the regime of tort liability with a contractual regime, where the parties, prior to the onset of medical services, set out the rules for liability and compensation once liability is established. The most obvious advantage of this system is that the contract mechanism will never end up with a set of rules that drives away patients who have a positive expected utility from receiving treatment. On the liability side, there could be a return to a gross negligence standard that restricts recovery to major and unexcused deviations from the applicable standard of care. On causation, the injured party would be required to show, by a clear preponderance of the evidence, the connection between the physician's misconduct and the patient's injury. On damages, recovery would be limited to some fraction of the total economic loss, similar to workers' compensation systems. Administratively, arbitration would replace litigation to reduce expenses. Any combination of these factors could bring down the expected costs of medical error to an affordable level.

I am not exactly sure how these contracts would play out if allowed. But that is part of the strength of using contractual devices. The current system runs haphazardly across specialties, across regions within a state, and across juries. That uncertainty itself is an economic cost that reduces or eliminates medical services. Using contracts allows both sides to circumvent these costly uncertainties. To this proposition, the common reply is that voluntary contracts will strip patients of all protection against mishap. This is possible, but not likely. Under competitive conditions, patients could easily decide that higher rates are worth some limited legal protection, especially when many individuals rely not on their own acumen, but on professional agents—employers, pension plans, and churches—to negotiate these deals for them. So informed parties can make the needed trade-offs. Health care providers can then let independent customers free-ride by offering deals similar to those given to plan members— taking care to guard against the adverse selection by those individually insured. Emergency room patients could be given the same deal as regular customers as a matter of course.

My sense is that this mechanism would outperform the current rules that derive from the *ex cathedra* statements of sitting judges who have little or no knowledge of how different liability regimes work. Indeed, whenever judges justify their rules by an appeal to notions of inequality of bargaining power or consumer ignorance, they only show their own woeful ignorance of how markets work. The inequality of bargaining power rationale is hopeless because it cannot explain how any contract is ever formed. The stronger party just asks for more and more concessions that the other side finds impossible to deny. But no agreement is ever that one-sided because people can and do say no as prices rise and terms become less attractive. The information story ignores the way in which intermediates and public sources can help fill the gap. Contracting is not perfect. But it works in area after area today. In the face of the repeated breakdowns of the medical malpractice system, we ignore this at our peril.

Statutory Reforms

Because of the failure to free up medical malpractice issues from the tort law, many proponents of malpractice reform today resort to legislative clout, and not contractual solutions, to reach more modest objectives. This clout should not be underestimated, for, unlike product manufacturers who face similar exposures, they tend to be in-state parties with lots of local political clout. But what have they wrought? The basic conclusion is this: There are lots of fancy reforms, but the only reform that has traction is a cap on damages, which could either apply only to pain and suffering, or could also extend to economic damages. These caps simply place a numerical maximum on the amount of damages that can be recovered. The number used for pain and suffering is often around $250,000. Total caps are usually for two or three times as much. Both figures are well below the multi-million judgments that could be obtained under earlier law. It was the cap on damages for noneconomic loss that was the major driver of increasing the access to physician care in Texas. And it is that same cap that has held down malpractice premiums in California.

The cap has these large effects for two reasons. The first is that it makes a huge difference in those large but infrequent cases. The $10 million noneconomic loss case is cut by 96 percent if a $250,000 cap is in place. In addition, the cap does not erode over time through inventive statutory readings by hostile judges; $250,000 remains the statutory figure, unless the statute adjusts it for inflation. Those two features make it easier to control insurance premiums, which tend to go down. But it hardly makes the cap ideal in principle. Noneconomic damages really matter in many cases. And it is hardly a triumph in reasoning to reduce the $1 million case and the $10 million case of pain and suffering award to the same $250,000 level. A system of damages that calls for proportionate reductions could preserve the difference between them. A contract system might adopt that approach, but it will not work as a legislative solution; it is too complicated to last.

As for the rest, shortening the statute of limitations will normally not do much good. Suits will be brought earlier and the defendant will agree to waive the statute if need be. Rules on joint and several liability kick in a small percentage of cases, and even then they do as much to switch damages among codefendants as to eliminate it. Reducing damages by collateral payments from health care plans can make a small dent in the system, but they do not touch either lost earnings or noneconomic damages. And so it goes. The politics that drive legislative reform do not get to the contractual ideal. But neither do the judges, which is why it is that medical malpractice will remain an open but not fatal wound for many years to come.

CONCLUSION

The basic story is not optimistic. To be sure, medical malpractice is not a first line social issue like taxes, bank regulation, or even health care reform. But it is an issue that matters for medical practitioners, at least for those physicians with high liability exposures. The current tort rules designed by judges miss the dynamics of any liability system. A strong dose of private contracting could help to keep matters measurable, but political and judicial resistance remains high. In consequence, the political struggles switch to statutory reforms of which a statutory cap on damages is the only one that matters. Adopted in some states and rejected in others, statutory reform promises to remain in the forefront of a struggle over medical malpractice liability that has already gone on far too long.

NOTES

1. For those who care about these things, see Patient Protection and Affordable Care Act, Pub. L. No. 111–148, 124 Stat. 119 (2010).

2. Amitabh Chandra, a noted Harvard economist, makes an upper-end estimate of $60BB/year for wasted treatment—about 3 percent of total health care spending, relative to actual direct costs of roughly $10 billion, or about half a percent of yearly medical spending. David Leonhardt, Medical Malpractice System, *The New York Times* (Sept. 22, 2009), available at www.nytimes.com/2009/09/23/business/economy/23leonhardt.html.

3. National Health Care Projections 2009–2019, available at https://146.123.140.205/NationalHealthExpendData/downloads/proj2009.pdf.

4. Tanya Albert Henry, "Defensive Medicine to Avoid Liability Lawsuits is Widespread," *American Medical News* (July 12, 2010), www.ama-assn.org/amednews/2010/07/12/prsb0712.htm.

5. James A. Comodeca, "Killing the Golden Goose by Evaluating Medical Care Through the Retroscope: Tort Reform From the Defense Perspective," 31 *Dayton Law Review* 207(2006): 214–15.

6. *See* Robert Guest, "Life is Expensive," *Economist*, May 30, 2009, at 12, 12 (estimating that Americans will spend $2.5 trillion on health care in 2009); Robert Pear, "Health spending in U.S. exceeds $2 trillion for the first time, *The New York Times* (Jan. 8, 2008), available at www.nytimes.com/2008/01/08/world/americas/08iht-health.4.9083459.html (showing health care spending first exceeded $2 trillion back in 2006).

7. David M. Studdert et al, "Claims, Errors, and Compensation Payments in Medical Malpractice Litigation," *New England Journal of Medicine* 354 (2006): 2024

8. Donald N. Dewees & Michael J. Trebilcock, "The Efficacy of the Tort System and its Alternatives: A Review of Empirical Evidence," Osgoode Hall Law Journal 30 (1992): 57.

9. Tunkl v. Regents of the University of California, 383 P.2d 441 (Cal. 1963).

10. Obstetrics & Gynecologists Ltd. v. Pepper, 693 P.2d 1259 (Nev. 1985).

11. Richard A. Epstein, "Medical Malpractice: The Case for Contract," 1 American Bar Foundation Research Journal 1 (1976): 87. For a similar view, see Patricia M. Danzon, *Medical Malpractice: Theory Evidence and Public Policy* (Cambridge: Harvard University Press, 1985). For a skeptical point of view, see Jennifer Arlen, *Contracting Over Malpractice Liability*, (NYU Law & Economics Research, Working Paper no. 08–12, 2008), *available at* http://papers.ssrn.com/sol3/papers.cfm?abstract_id=1105368.

7

LESSONS FROM STATE HEALTH REFORMS

Roger Stark, MD

S INCE THE FAILURE OF HillaryCare at the national
level in the early 1990s a number of states have made
attempts at implementing health care reform of
their own. Each of these has been based on some form of
government-managed system, generally including an open-
ended taxpayer funding commitment, combined with a
generous set of mandated benefits.

In each case, these programs failed to achieve their policy
goals and have often proved unsustainable as originally
enacted. Naturally, backers of these health care programs
are reluctant to talk about their original ideas once they
have failed, so past state efforts at health care reform tend
to be forgotten. This is unfortunate, because the hard-won
experiences of states should have influenced the debate over
federal health care reform.

Roger Stark is a health care policy analyst for the Washington Policy Center for
Health Care.

This study includes a review of six states, Washington, Oregon, Tennessee, Hawaii, Massachusetts, and Maine, that enacted government-managed health care reform plans; two states, Wisconsin and California, where such plans were proposed but failed to pass; and three states that took a different approach. These three states, Florida, Georgia and Indiana, enacted reforms that move decision-making about health care to the individual, work with market forces, and create voluntary incentives that increase choice and expand access to health care coverage.

GOVERNMENT-MANAGED STATE REFORM PLANS

Washington: The Washington State Health Plan

In 1993, Washington had approximately 600,000 uninsured residents, which represented about 11 percent of the population. That year the legislature passed sweeping health care reform legislation, called the Washington State Health Plan, in an effort to reduce the number of uninsured and make health coverage more affordable.

The basis of the program was to require all state residents not in Medicare to join a managed competition plan. The primary goal of the program was to provide universal coverage for all Washington residents. The policy elements of the program included:

1. Price controls in the form of state-imposed caps on insurance premiums;
2. Statewide community ratings and universal access;

3. New mandates on employers and individuals;
4. A guaranteed-issue law, and;
5. Increased emphasis on public health and prevention.

The plan added a powerful new state bureaucracy, raised taxes, added more mandates and restrictions on employers and individuals, and gave state government vastly expanded control over health care.

The consequences of the plan were devastating. Fourteen health insurance carriers left the state, and the few remaining insurance companies were forced to raise their rates by up to 40 percent. The number of uninsured in Washington rose by 20 percent, as people were forced to drop policies they could no longer afford. The state began attracting sick people from all over the country because of the guaranteed-issue provision.

The guaranteed-issue law required insurers to sell their product to anyone, regardless of medical risk or pre-existing health conditions. One insurance company received a polite letter from one satisfied policyholder. She had purchased an insurance policy during her recent pregnancy and, now that her baby was born, she no longer needed the policy and was dropping her coverage. She assured the company she would certainly choose it again when she needed to pay for medical care in the future.[1]

The community-rating law required premiums charged by an insurance company to be an average of all premiums (for sick and healthy, young and old, etc.) in a given region. Exceptions were allowed for some factors, such as age, but the required community-rating "bands" (legal limits on how much the cost of coverage could vary) worked as a price control. The restriction kept insurers from accurately setting monthly premiums to reflect the real risk involved in selling someone a particular insurance policy.

Together, community-rating and guaranteed-issue rules created two perverse incentives. First, they encouraged healthy people to avoid buying health insurance, since the average rate they would pay was far higher than what they would pay in an unregulated market. Second, they encouraged people to wait until they got sick before buying insurance.

Community rating makes the price less than what a sick person would pay in an unregulated market and guaranteed issue forces insurance companies to sell a sick person a policy, after a waiting period, without taking all the medical risks involved into account. These rules result in higher health insurance prices for everyone.

By 1994, it was obvious the plan was not working and a citizen revolt occurred at the voting booths. The governing party in the legislature lost its majority, and the governor who had signed the reform plan was forced to approve a repeal of the program, in order to avoid an embarrassing vote on the issue through a popular initiative.[2]

While most elements of the 1992 reform plan were repealed, Washington's health insurance market never fully recovered. This is in part because the guaranteed-issue law, though modified, remains in place, the market is burdened by more than fifty-seven state-imposed mandates; and the state levies a special tax on all insurance policies sold in Washington.

Supporters of the Washington State Health Plan said when it was passed that it would provide universal coverage and lower health care costs, but the plan failed in both respects. Instead, the legacy of the Washington State Health Plan is an insurance market burdened with costly regulations, particularly the high number of mandates, the guaranteed-issue law and the community-rating requirement. Today in-state health costs are higher than ever, and the uninsured rate is no lower than when the plan was first proposed.

Oregon: The Oregon Health Plan

The Oregon Health Plan was created in 1994 and by the following year it had 132,000 enrollees. The plan offered coverage to all Oregon residents under age sixty-five who could not afford individual plans or were not covered by their employers, but whose income was not low enough to make them eligible for Medicaid.

The plan did, however, require people in the state Medicaid program to join a managed care plan. Consequently the cost of Oregon Medicaid grew from $750 million a biennium before the Oregon Health Plan started, to $1.7 billion in the first biennium after the program was introduced.

Oregon lawmakers soon found they could not afford the rising costs of the plan they had created. Similarly, insurance carriers in the state dropped out of the Oregon Health Plan because the state's low reimbursement rates made participation economically impractical for them.[3]

By 2004, because of the high cost of the program, Oregon stopped taking new enrollees and total enrollment fell to only

18,000 people. In 2008, Oregon held a statewide lottery in an effort to control spiraling costs while adding 6,000 new enrollees.[4] In the process, Oregon Health Plan officials gave up on trying to provide universal coverage.

Oregon lawmakers learned that the ambitious plan enacted in 1994 was fiscally unsustainable, and the program has survived only by being sharply cut back. In the long run, the Oregon Health Plan has failed to reduce significantly the number of uninsured, or to control rising health care costs in the state, as supporters had promised.

Tennessee: The TennCare Plan

In 1994, lawmakers in Tennessee created TennCare, a state health plan based on eleven state-run managed care organizations (MCOs) offering unlimited doctor visits, hospital stays, and a prescription drug benefit. As part of TennCare, the state required 800,000 Medicaid recipients to move into the MCOs, and then added 500,000 uninsured or high-risk individuals to the program. In 1995, Tennessee officials were forced by rising costs to close the program to new enrollments.

Because of rapidly escalating program costs, doctors working under TennCare were financially squeezed until 1999 when they lobbied strongly to receive a certain percentage of the state money paid to MCOs. This new mandate highlighted the fact that MCOs were failing to control costs and provide adequate medical care. Three of the original MCOs soon went out of business, and the state itself nearly went bankrupt, even though the federal government was paying two-thirds of program costs. In 2005, state officials dropped 160,000 people who were not Medicaid eligible from the program.[5]

With TennCare in financial shambles, the legislature enacted Cover Tennessee in 2006, in an effort to provide coverage for people that state officials had barred from the original plan. Cover Tennessee is designed for enrollees who earn less than 250 percent of the federal poverty level. It provided mandated first dollar coverage (benefits that are not subject to a deductible or copayment), but no catastrophic coverage above $25,000 per year. Only $15,000 of this $25,000 can go toward hospital bills. Cover Tennessee is proving no more successful than TennCare because the new program suffers from similar structural weaknesses: state-management, lack of enrollee control over benefits, and numerous top-down mandates.[6]

Hawaii: The Individual Mandate Plan and Universal Coverage for Children

Hawaii has had an employer mandate in place since 1974 when two percent of the population was uninsured.[7] Currently, employers must either provide a set level of health care benefits, as defined by law, to their employees, or pay a special tax into a state-managed fund. The program is a real-world example of the "pay-or-play" approach to health care reform that has been considered by many other states. After more than thirty years with a universal state-imposed health care mandate, Hawaii continues to experience rising health care costs, and today has an uninsured rate close to 10 percent.

In 2007, Hawaii's Democratic legislature passed universal health insurance for children up to age 19. The bill was signed into law by Governor Linda Lingle, a Republican. The goal was to provide health insurance to an estimated 3,500 uninsured children who were not Medicaid-eligible but were from families that could not afford private insurance at $55 per month. Keiki Care (Keiki is Hawaiian for child) was funded by state taxpayers plus a 50 percent match from Hawaii Medical Service Association (HMSA), the independent private licensee of Blue Cross and Blue Shield in the state.[8]

Within seven months the governor closed the program because of a skyrocketing state deficit ($162 million for 2008) and because 85 percent of the 2000 children enrolled had dropped their private insurance to join Keiki Care. HMSA found a 95 percent drop in its private insurance customers which confirmed a "crowd out" of lower-income kids by children of families that could afford private insurance.[9]

The state is now encouraging families with incomes less than 300 percent of the federal poverty level ($73,000 for a family of four) to enroll their children in the State-Children's Health Insurance Plan (S-CHIP).

Massachusetts: The Health Connector Plan

The Massachusetts legislature passed comprehensive health care reform in the spring of 2006 to deal with escalating costs as well as 550,000 uninsured people (8.6 percent of the population), and to ensure that all state residents have health care coverage.[10] Proponents said a major benefit of the plan would be universal coverage, and that the state's uninsured population would be reduced to zero.

Basic to the plan is a mandate that every resident between the ages of eighteen and sixty-four purchase a state-defined health insurance policy. This is combined with a mandate on all employers with more than ten workers to provide state-defined health care coverage, or pay a special tax of $295 per employee into a state fund. The state created a Health Connector program for the individual and small group markets to help residents and employers buy the state-mandated coverage.

The state provides subsidies on a sliding scale for residents with incomes of less than 300 percent of the federal poverty level. Residents with incomes below the federal poverty level pay nothing; the state provides them with subsidized coverage.

The Health Connector takes over the role of private-sector insurance agents by matching individuals with state-approved health plans. Although the program did not add new mandates, plans purchased through the Connector must include all existing state mandates for medical services and coverage. The Connector also increased the risk pool and enhanced the portability of insurance. Individuals are able to retain their Connector-based coverage as they leave the workforce or move from job to job.[11]

The Massachusetts plan was the template for the recently passed federal health care reform. Both programs contain individual and employer mandates, an insurance exchange with taxpayer subsidies, increased government regulation of the health insurance industry including community rating and guaranteed issue, and an expansion of Medicaid to 300 percent of the federal poverty level.

So what has happened in Massachusetts?

By December 2008, approximately 383,000 people who previously had no insurance were covered by the state plan.[12] Unfortunately, the majority of these residents are in an entitlement program called Commonwealth Care that is partially or wholly subsidized by state taxpayers.

Individual private plans are not selling well. In April 2007, the Health Connector Board was forced to exempt 20 percent of the uninsured from the individual mandate and increased the subsidy to low-income residents. Proponents of the Massachusetts plan are no longer saying it will provide universal coverage.

The plan has resulted in a dramatic increase in demand for medical services, to the point where primary care doctors are in short supply. Waiting times to see a family physician are up to 100 days in parts of Massachusetts while the number of practices accepting new patients has plummeted.[13]

Costs have skyrocketed with early budget over-runs of 30 percent, while overall health care costs in the state continue to rise at 8 percent annually. Originally, backers provided no budget beyond the first three years of the program, and the governor asked for an additional $869 million in 2009. He admits that number may be low and could reach as high as $1.1 billion. In the next decade there is a predicted cost over-run of $4 billion. At various times, the governor has proposed tax increases in an effort to shore up the program.[14] To control costs further, the legislature is considering cutting payments to doctors and going to global reimbursement schemes, increasing the special tax on employers (currently $295 a year), and imposing additional regulations on insurers and drug companies. An additional $1.00-per-pack cigarette tax has already been added.

There is no proposal to decrease state-imposed mandates on individual insurance plans, and consequently Massachusetts insurance carriers are unable to offer low-cost plans.

Massachusetts now has the highest health insurance rates in the country,[15] yet all major insurance carriers reported losses of millions of dollars for the first quarter of 2010. The companies want to increase rates, but the governor has imposed a price control on the industry capped at a 7.7 percent rate increase per year.[16]

Maine: The Dirigo Health Plan

Maine lawmakers enacted a sweeping health care reform plan, Dirigo Health, in 2005 with the intention of containing health care costs, insuring broad access, and improving quality. *Dirigo*, which is Latin for "I direct" or "I lead," is Maine's state motto.

Supporters predicted a total enrollment of 130,000 people by 2009. Dirigo was initially available to uninsured individuals and to business owners with fewer than fifty employees, which included 90 percent of Maine businesses.

The plan includes a guaranteed-issue requirement and both low-and high-deductible plans are available. The overall program is run through Anthem, a private insurance carrier.

Funding comes from individual enrollees, a onetime $53 million state "grant," and federal subsidies for people earning less than 200 percent of the federal poverty level. Employers must pay 60 percent of premium costs and the state pays on a sliding scale for people earning between 200 percent and 300 percent of the poverty level. Other premium costs are borne by individuals. Insurance companies are assessed a special tax of four percent on all health insurance policies sold in the state. The Dirigo plan also includes additional Certificate of Need restrictions, thus making it difficult for doctors and clinics to provide new medical services.[17] (Some states and federal jurisdictions require a "Certificate of Need" before proposed health care acquisitions, expansions, or new facilities are allowed.)

Like other state-directed plans, Dirigo has not provided the level of health coverage promised by advocates, nor has it succeeded in controlling costs. In fact, the opposite has occurred. After the first few years the program proved unsustainable. In an effort to save it, lawmakers are considering a new employer mandate (based on the pay-or-play model used in Hawaii), a separate state high-risk pool, and imposing more Medicaid price controls. Also, instead of using the private insurance company, Anthem, Maine is considering administering the program itself.

In April 2008, the legislature enacted a tax increase on soft drinks, beer and wine, and added a 1.8 percent tax on health care claims. Revenue from the new taxes was intended to shore up the Dirigo program. However, Maine residents voted overwhelmingly to repeal the tax in November 2008.[18] At present, fewer than 3,500 previously uninsured people are covered under Maine's "public option" insurance plan. Costs to Maine's taxpayers have exceeded $155 million through fiscal year 2009, while premium costs have skyrocketed 74 percent in four years.[19] The program has gone through periods of being unable to accept new enrollees.[20] Dirigo's website has carried a notice, "We are not offering subsidized coverage to new members at this time due to lack of funding."[21] Dirigo administrators are urging Maine residents to contact the governor and lawmakers in Augusta to express their views about the uncertain future of the program.[22]

STATE-MANAGED PLANS RECENTLY PROPOSED, BUT NOT ADOPTED

Wisconsin: The Healthy Wisconsin Plan

The "Healthy Wisconsin" plan was proposed in 2008 and would have begun in 2009, but it failed to pass the legislature. The plan would have mandated coverage for all state residents not enrolled in an existing government program such as Medicaid and Medicare. The framework for the program was a governor-appointed board that would negotiate payment rates with doctors and solicit uniform health plan bids from insurance carriers. The board was to be composed of eleven members, five representing labor unions, four representing businesses other than insurance carriers, and two named by farming organizations.

Like previous state health care plans, Healthy Wisconsin promised universal coverage while lowering costs. As its promoters describe it: "Healthy Wisconsin will for the first time guarantee that all Wisconsinites get the same high quality health care that our state legislators have had for years, while being affordable for Wisconsin families."[23]

The plan's funding was based on a new 14.5 percent payroll tax, 10.5 percent of which would be levied on employers, and 4 percent directly on employees. In practice, of course, all 14.5 percent of the tax would have been paid by workers, since for employers, paying the tax would simply become part of the routine cost of hiring a new employee. As such, 10.5 percent of the economic value of hiring a new worker would be paid to the state government, instead of going to the worker in the form of salary or other compensation.

If it had been passed, Healthy Wisconsin's new 14.5 percent payroll tax would have added to the existing 15.3 percent tax workers already pay to fund Social Security and Medicare. The combined 29.8 percent tax would have ranked Wisconsin as highest in the nation in payroll taxes.

Supporters said that much of the tax on employment would have been offset by employers not having to buy separate insurance coverage for their workers.

The first year's budget estimate for the Healthy Wisconsin plan was $15.2 billion, which would have essentially doubled the state budget. Out-of-pocket expenses for individuals would have been limited to $3,000 a year and there would have been no co-payments or charges for preventative and pediatric care. Even though the plan was enormous in scope, it was offered as a last minute amendment to the state budget, with only one rushed hearing.[24]

Interestingly, the politically powerful teachers' union was made exempt from the plan, and a substantial loophole allowed other labor unions to opt out of the program. The broad exemption had the effect of muting labor opposition to the plan.

Even its proponents acknowledged that Healthy Wisconsin's taxes would have potentially caused job losses for up to 8,000 mostly low-paid workers. They claimed that a family earning less than $50,000 a year would potentially have saved money, and that a family earning more than $50,000 a year would have spent more on health care. The secretary of the administration was charged with containing costs if individuals in the plan spent more on health care than the national average.

California: Coverage for All Californians

In 2007, Governor Arnold Schwarzenegger, working with the state assembly leadership, proposed a sweeping health care reform plan. The plan was based on a mandate on individuals requiring everyone not in Medicare or MediCal (California's Medicaid program) to purchase health insurance, plus a mandate on employers to either provide worker health insurance or pay an additional business tax of 10 percent to the state (the pay-or-play model). The employer mandate applied to all firms with more than nine employees. The plan also included a guaranteed-issue provision under which insurers were required to sell their product to anyone who asked for it, regardless of medical risk.[25]

Funding was to be provided by an additional 6 percent payroll tax, a 2 percent tax on physicians and a 4 percent tax on hospitals, plus an additional $1.50- to $2.00-per-pack tax on cigarettes. The new state payroll tax would have been added to the 15.3 percent tax workers already pay in federal Social Security and Medicaid taxes. State officials planned to secure $5 billion more by expanding the definition of the MediCal program, making it eligible to receive increased federal funding. Total cost of the plan was estimated at $14 billion per year.[26]

From the start, the governor's plan faced serious political and economic obstacles. Even without a new payroll tax and employer mandate, California ranked fourth from the bottom in a national poll of "best states to do business."[27] Also, in 2007 California faced a budget deficit of $14 billion, making many lawmakers reluctant to take on new, permanent financial responsibilities.

In December 2007, the California Assembly approved the new health care plan on a party line vote, with Democrats voting in favor and most Republicans, despite the governor's support, opposed. The following month, however, the Senate Health Care Committee rejected the plan, ending prospects for passage.[28]

The rejection of broad-based universal health care plans in Wisconsin and California indicates that enthusiasm for government-managed reform may be fading among state lawmakers. The proposals in these two states contained most of the elements of classic single-payer-style plans: universal coverage, new payroll and business taxes, expansion of the state Medicaid program, new mandates on employers and individuals, and central management through a state-appointed board or agency.

Fifteen years of debate and trial at the state level indicate that this policy approach was successful in expanding access to affordable health care or in reducing the number of uninsured.

A DIFFERENT APPROACH: STATES USING INDIVIDUAL CHOICE AND MARKET COMPETITION TO LOWER COSTS

While several states attempted, with little success, to reduce costs and help the uninsured by enacting versions of single-payer-style plans, leaders in three states took a different approach. Lawmakers in Florida, Georgia, and Indiana have enacted reforms that reduce costs by trimming state regulations, promoting individual control over health care spending and tapping competitive market forces.

These plans do not promise universal coverage. Instead, they direct reform policies toward people who need the most help in getting health coverage: low-income families, the chronically ill, and the uninsured.

Florida: The Cover Florida Plan, Promoting Market Competition

The Cover Florida plan was enacted in May 2008 to provide health care coverage for the 20 percent of Floridians who are uninsured. The plan is voluntary and is available to people earning less than 300 percent of the federal poverty level and who have been uninsured for more than six months.[29] Cover Florida lowers monthly premium costs for each enrollee to between $100 and $150 by streamlining regulations and legalizing economical, low-cost health coverage.

The state plan has sparked a competition among private insurers to offer attractively priced plans which, under Cover Florida, are exempt from Florida's fifty health care mandates. National studies show that state mandates add 15 percent to 25 percent to the cost of health care coverage.[30]

While free of most top-down regulations, the plans must include basic preventative and primary care services, such as screening, office visits, outpatient and inpatient surgery, urgent care, prescription drugs, durable medical equipment and diabetic supplies.[31] To keep the plans affordable, they do not cover prolonged hospital stays or specialty care. Insurers must offer policyholders an option for catastrophic care, and may charge a higher monthly premium for this higher level of coverage.

Cover Florida uses a fifteen-member oversight board to negotiate rates and handle claims for the state's small businesses (those with fewer than fifty employees). Again, the plan is voluntary. Small business owners are not required to participate, and may use competitive offerings in the private market to design their own health care benefit plan if they wish. The Cover Florida plan avoids centralized government management of people's health care. Instead, the plan taps the participation of private insurance companies that agree to accept all enrollees, and uses market competition to lower costs and expand access to coverage for the uninsured. The plan has been successful at increasing affordable options for Floridians seeking health coverage. To date, nine insurers have submitted proposals to participate in the program.[32]

Georgia: Access to Health Coverage through Low-Cost HSAs

Georgia passed a law in May 2008 that encourages the voluntary use of portable, low-cost Health Savings Accounts (HSAs) to provide health care coverage.[33] The law went into effect in January 2009.

Under the plan, residents are able to deduct all of the cost of HSA-related insurance premiums from their income when calculating their state income tax liability. The result is an immediate 6 percent reduction in the cost of health coverage for individuals.[34]

Small business owners (those with fifty or fewer employees) who offer HSA coverage to their employees receive a $250 tax credit per worker. Under previous law many small employers could not afford to provide an employee health benefit, or had dropped benefits they had provided in the past. Under the new plan a small business owner with, say, ten workers, who provided them with HSA coverage would see an immediate reduction of $2,500 a year state taxes.

In addition, Georgia lawmakers repealed state and local taxes on HSA-based insurance premiums, thus further lowering the market price of HSA plans. The legislature estimates that Georgia's consumer-friendly approach reduced the cost of HSA-based insurance plans by $146 million a year, lowered taxes for employers by $64.8 million a year, and saved workers $6.7 million a year.[35] The reduction in regulations and taxes is expected to ultimately expand access to affordable health coverage to 500,000 uninsured Georgia residents.[36]

Indiana: The Healthy Indiana Plan

The "Healthy Indiana Plan" began in January 2008. It is limited to the first 120,000 applicants who have had no health care insurance for at least six months and who earn less than 200 percent of the federal poverty level.

The program has two parts: a state-funded HSA plus a high-deductible catastrophic health insurance plan. Low-income individuals can use money placed in the HSA to pay for preventative care and routine health services. If funds in the HSA prove insufficient, benefits from the catastrophic health plan are then available to cover major medical costs.

To keep the HSA plans affordable, an individual's contribution is limited to no more than 5 percent of gross family income.[37] The federal government granted Indiana a Medicaid waiver to allow state officials to lower HSA costs for low-income families.[38] The legislature enacted a forty-four-cent increase in the state cigarette tax to help fund the program.

The main advantage of Healthy Indiana is that it puts low-income residents in charge of their own health benefit, rather than placing them in the position of being passive recipients of a traditional welfare program. Program participants are not restricted to public health clinics or to public health hospitals. Using their HSA funds, they can choose their own doctors and make decisions about their own health needs without facing the barriers commonly imposed by public assistance programs. In addition, funds placed in the HSA become the recipients' private property, thus helping low-income families rise out of poverty.

Although Indiana's plan has been very popular, it is uncertain whether HSAs will meet the new federal "qualified coverage" standard.[39]

CONCLUSION

In consideration of lessons learned from alternative health systems and previous health reforms, policymakers need not restrict their analyses to other countries. In fact, a number of conclusions can be drawn from the American experience—from our own states with failed government-managed health care plans, and from our states that have taken a market-oriented approach.

The first and most obvious lesson is that the health care problem cannot be solved with more government control.

In each case studied, increased government management of health care led to higher costs, lower accessibility, and, in many cases, fewer people being covered.

Second, the conclusion that flows from this experience is that top-down mandatory approaches do not work. State leaders should not force either mandated benefits or mandated enrollment upon their constituents. Mandated benefits restrict choice in the type and amount of insurance a person can purchase, without taking account of an individual's personal situation or life needs. Mandating individual enrollment has not been effective, as demonstrated by Hawaii's experience. After more than thirty years of imposing the broadest individual mandate possible—that all state residents must have health coverage—Hawaii's rate of uninsured is higher today than when the law passed.

Third, price controls do not lower costs, but they do lead to rationing and an increase in the number of uninsured. Community rating, guaranteed issue, and insurance premium caps are efforts by policymakers to limit rising costs by simply banning price increases. But, as political leaders have learned through the centuries, price controls never work. Normal prices are set by the interaction of supply and demand. No amount of political will or government power can change this basic economic principle.

A fourth lesson from the states is that policymakers should not promise the public universal coverage. A common theme among states that imposed mandatory health care reform is that, in return for accepting government management of health care, all citizens would receive coverage. In every case, from Maine to Washington, government-managed systems failed to achieve universal coverage. They often had the opposite effect as increased taxes and regulations reduced competition among insurers drove up premiums, and led many individuals and employers to drop their existing coverage.

Rather than focusing on universal, top-down approaches, policymakers should recognize that the most important person in any health care reform is the individual. It is incumbent upon state governments to provide a free and open market so people can access medical care in an efficient and cost-effective manner.

Dr. Robert Moffit of the Heritage Foundation succinctly outlined the key tests that state legislators should apply to any health care reform proposal:

- The new plan should focus on changing the existing system—not merely expanding existing programs;
- It should make individual patients the key decision makers;
- It should create dependable coverage not subject to the whim of the political process;
- It should limit the role of government;
- The value of the new plan must be much greater to the patient than to anyone else in the system, such as regulators or politicians;
- It should comply with existing federal law.[40]

States that implement individual-based reforms have achieved positive results by not promising a utopian vision of universal access. They recognize there will always be a role for tax-funded safety net health programs, but that with the right public policies, most people can access affordable health coverage through a competitive private market. In a functioning health care market, prices, innovation and services would be determined by voluntary transactions between patients and providers, with government regulations providing necessary public safety and consumer protections.

The needs and situation of each state are unique, yet the principles of successful health care reform apply across all states. Looking ahead, lawmakers can benefit from a close examination of reform efforts in other states, and adopt a policy approach that will lower health care costs and increase access for all people.

NOTES

1. Once this story became known in the legislature, lawmakers eased the guaranteed-issue law to allow insurers to require a nine-month waiting period before a newly purchased insurance policy would cover a pre-existing medical condition.

2. Robert Cihak, MD, Bob Williams, and Peter J. Ferrara, "The Rise and Repeal of the Washington State Health Plan: Lessons for America's State Legislators," June 11, 1997, at www.heritage.org/research/health care/bg1121.cfm.

3. Alan Katz, "The Oregon Health Insurance Lottery," Health Care Reform Blog, March 4, 2008, at www.alankatz.wordpress.com/2008/03/04/the-oregon-health-insurance-lottery.

4. Sarah Skidmore, "Prize in Oregon Lottery is Health Insurance," *Seattle Times*, March 2, 2008.

5. "HillaryCare in Tennessee, the Disaster that Might Have Been for the Entire Country," Review and Outlook, *Wall Street Journal*, December 6, 2004, at www.opinionjournal.com/editorial/feature.html?id=110005987.

6. Drew Johnson, "Cover Tennessee is No Magic Cure for the Uninsured," Tennessee Center for Policy Research, April 28, 2008, at www.tennesseepolicy.org/main/article.php?article_id=709.

7. "Too Many Residents Lack Health Insurance," editorial page, *Honolulu Star-Bulletin*, October 18, 2005, at www.starbulletin.com/ 2005/10/18/editorial/editorials.html.

8. www.galen.org/component,8/action,show_content/id,13/blog _id,1108 /category_id,8/type,33/, accessed July 20, 2010.

9. www.heartland.org/publications/budget%20tax/article/24294/ Hawaii_Drops_Universal_Childrens_Health_Care_Plan.html, accessed July 20, 2010.

10. Pam Belluck, "Massachusetts Sets Health Plan for Nearly All," *New York Times*, April 15, 2006.

11. David Hyman "The Massachusetts health plan: The good, the bad, and the ugly," *Policy Analysis*, The Cato Institute, June 28, 2007, at www.cato.org/pub_display.php?pub_id=8431.

12. Sharon K. Long, Allison Cook, and Karen Stockley, "Health Insurance Coverage in Massachusetts: Estimates from the 2008 Massachusetts Health Insurance Survey," Urban Institute, December 18, 2008.

13. Liz Kowalczyk, "Across Massachusetts, Wait to See Doctors Grows," *Boston Globe*, September 22, 2008.

14. "The Price of Romney Care," Editorial Page, *Wall Street Journal*, July 29, 2008.

15. Joseph Rago, "The Massachusetts Health Care 'Train Wreck,' " *Wall Street Journal*, July 7, 2010.

16. Naftali Bendavid, "Massachusetts Race Highlights Health Care," *Wall Street Journal*, June 14, 2010.

17. Universal Health Care Initiative—Maine, *The Equity Sector*, March 9, 2005.

18. "John Kartch and Kelly Cobb, Mainers Vote Overwhelmingly to Repeal Dirigo Health Tax," *Americans for Tax Reform*, November 6, 2008.

19. Tarren Bragdon, "A series of Unfortunate Events: Dirigo— Maine's "Public Option" is a Costly Failure," *Crisis to Cure*, no. 3, (June 30, 2009).

20. Pam Belluck, "As Health Plans Falter, Maine Explores Changes," *New York Times*, May 30, 2007.

21. Dirigo Health, main page, at www.dirigohealth.maine.gov/ accessed July 30, 2008.

22. Ibid.

23. "Healthy Wisconsin, Your Choice, Your Plan," Institute for One Wisconsin, at www.healthywisconsin.net, accessed July 30, 2008.

24. Author interview with Christian Schneider, Health Care Analyst, Wisconsin Policy Research Institute, May 13, 2008.

25. "The Governor's Health Care Plan," at www.fixourhealthcare.ca.gov/plan, accessed June 26, 2008.

26. Jeff Emanuel, "California Health Insurance Plan a Bad Idea," *Human Events*, December 20, 2007.

27. Chris Atkins and Curtis S. Dubay, "State Business Tax Climate Index Ranking (Fifth Edition)," by Background Paper no. 57, National Tax Foundation, 2008, at www.taxfoundation.org/research/show/22658.html.

28. "State Watch, California Senate Health Care Committee Rejects Plan to Overhaul State Health Care System," at www.kaisernetwork.org/DailyReports/repindex.cfm?DRID=50084.

29. Doug Trapp, "Florida Passes Bill to Boost Private Health Coverage for Uninsured," *amednews.com*, June 2, 2008, at www.ama-assn.org/amednews/2008/06/02/gvsb0602.htm.

30. Paul Guppy, "How Mandates Increase Costs and Reduce Access to Health Care Coverage," Policy Brief, Washington Policy Center, June 2002, at www.washingtonpolicy.org/Centers/healthcare/policy brief/02_guppy_mandates. html.

31. "Cover Florida, Statement by Governor Crist regarding release of intent to negotiate for Cover Florida plan," Office of the Governor, June 2008, at www.flgov.com/cover_florida.

32. "Nine insurers seek to 'Cover Florida,'" The Buzz, *St. Petersburg Times*, August 18, 2008, at www.blogs.tampabay.com/buzz/2008/08/nine-insurers-s.html.

33. H.B. 977, "State Insurance Premium Taxes; Certain High Deductible Health Plans; Exempt," Georgia General Assembly, signed May 7, 2008, www.legis.state.ga.us/legis/2007_08/sum/hb977.htm.

34. "Georgia Passes HRA/HSA Health Insurance Reforms," National Center for Policy Analysis, May 2008, at NCPA.org, "Georgia HSA tax break bill signed into law," by Jerry Geisel, Business Insurance, May 8, 2008, at www.businessinsurance.com/cgi-bin/news.pl?id=12918.

35. Ron Bachman, "Impact of Insuring 500,000 Georgians Previously Uninsured," senior fellow, Center for Health Transformation,

May 9, 2008, at www.healthtransformation.net/galleries/wp-consumer ism/TheEconomicImpactofHB977.pdf.

36. Ibid.

37. Healthy Indiana Plan, *Evansville (IN) Courier & Press*, January 1, 2008.

38. "HHS approves Medicaid waiver to create new Indiana Health Plan for uninsured Hoosiers," press release, U.S. Department of Health and Human Services, December 14, 2007, at www.hhs.gov/news/press/2007pres/12/pr20071214a.html.

39. Thomas Cheplick, "Obamacare Threatens Indiana's HSA Program," *Health Care News*, June 2010.

40. Robert E. Moffit, PhD, "State Health Reform: Six Key Tests," Web Memo no. 1900, The Heritage Foundation, April 23, 2008, at www.heritage.org/Research/healthcare/wm1900.cfm.

8

GOVERNMENT CONTROL ON ACCESS TO CARE: CANADA'S EXPERIENCE

Nadeem Esmail

ANADA'S GOVERNMENT-RUN health insurance system is often held to be a guiding light for health care reform in the United States. Statements vilifying private insurers and allusions revealing the ultimate desire for a single payer system by government officials—from the president to congressional leaders—are easy to document. Unfortunately, those who propose adopting a Canadian-style health care program often ignore or misrepresent the realities of putting government in charge of the health insurance system. Canadians, on the other hand, are made aware of the consequences of government control over health care on a daily basis.

Before discussing the consequences of government management of Canada's health care system, it is worthwhile to clarify the role of government in Canada's health insurance and delivery systems.

Economist and analyst Nadeem Esmail is a Senior Fellow at the Fraser Institute.

With respect to insurance, Canada's provincial governments are monopoly providers of insurance and funding for "medically necessary"[1] physician and hospital services. This is an important departure from the role of government in every other developed nation where private insurance and payment for physician and hospital services are not prohibited.

Conversely, provincial governments offer insurance for dental care and out of hospital pharmaceuticals for only select segments of the population, such as seniors and low-income individuals, leaving many Canadians to either pay out of pocket or rely on their employer or themselves for private dental and pharmaceutical insurance coverage.

With respect to the provision of health care services, the vast majority of hospital care is delivered in public hospitals with privately owned surgical clinics playing a small role.[2] Physicians, on the other hand, are primarily private contractors, although they receive almost all of their monies from their provincial government insurance program due to prohibitions on private funding of medically necessary physician care.

While there are some exceptions in provinces like Quebec and British Columbia, this is the basic structure of the Canadian health care system. What should be clear is the dominant role that government plays in both the funding and delivery of health care. And that dominant role means that government decides how much will be spent on health care and how much access to health care will be restricted and rationed.

On the spending side, Canada's governments have been generous with the amount of tax dollars committed to health care. Since 1999, the first year for which measures of age-adjusted health care expenditures in nations that maintain universal-access health insurance programs are available,[3] Canada's has ranked among the three most expensive universal-access health insurance systems in the developed world. Health expenditures in the most recent year for which comparable data are available are shown in Figure 8.1. And this recent spending record is not a departure from the past: government health care expenditures in Canada have been growing faster than the economy as a whole for many years.[4]

Canada's high level of spending and spending growth might be considered irresponsible, and certainly indicate that government control has not been an effective solution to the high cost of health care. Importantly, for six of Canada's ten provinces, government health care expenditures are on track to consume half of available revenues by 2034. For two of those provinces, including Canada's largest province by population, expenditures are on pace to reach this milestone by 2014 or earlier.[5]

This trend analysis does not capture the full story of Canada's future health spending problem. Critically, Canada's elderly (who tend to be more costly to care for than their younger counterparts) are expected to constitute a much larger share of the population in the future. This change in Canada's demographic makeup will continue to increase the amount of revenue needed to fund Medicare expenditures. It has been estimated that the difference between the

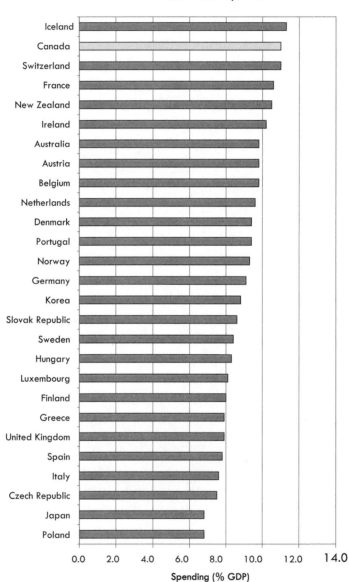

FIGURE 8.1

Age-adjusted health spending (% GDP) in select OECD countries, 2005

Spending (% GDP)

Source: Nadeem Esmail and Michael Walker, "How Good is Canadian Health Care?" (Vancouver: Fraser Institute, 2009 Report).

stream of promised benefits and the expected future stream of revenues—the unfunded liability of Medicare—was $364 billion in 2004,[6] the latest year for which the estimate is available. This compares to government health expenditures of $84.6 billion that year.[7] Notably, Medicare's unfunded liability grew by 21 percent between 2000 and 2004, from $301.5 billion to $364.0 billion.[8]

Despite the significant and growing health care expenditures by Canada's governments, Canadians have been provided with remarkably poor access to health care services. Perhaps the best known measure of this is the long wait times Canadians must endure for nearly all forms of government funded medical care. For example, in 2009 the average Canadian could expect to wait 16.1 weeks from mandatory referral by a general practitioner to treatment by a specialist.[9] (See Figure 8.2.) Of that 16.1 weeks waiting, 8.2 weeks were to see the specialist in the first place prior to treatment.[10]

The growth in wait times tells an even more troubling story. Although Canada's provinces have increased health care spending considerably, the total wait time in 2009 was 73 percent longer than in 1993 (Figure 8.2).[11] Statistical analyses of wait times and health expenditures show a clearly dysfunctional relationship in which increases in taxpayer resources committed to health care are either unrelated to or positively related with the length of time Canadians must wait for medical treatment.[12]

Notably, wait times for medical care in Canada vary depending on the risk of death from the underlying condition. In 2009 for example, the median wait times for cancer treatment by a radiation or medical oncologist were about five weeks from referral by a general practitioner while the median wait time for neurosurgery stretched to 32.9 weeks and to 33.7 weeks for orthopedic surgery.[13] (See Figure 8.2.) Put simply, the burden of waiting for medical care in Canada falls heavily on those who are waiting for treatment of painful and debilitating but not necessarily fatal conditions.

While the wait times for specialist care and elective medical treatments are those most often quoted and discussed in the media, there are many other wait times that plague

FIGURE 8.2
Wait Times for Medical Care in Canada,
GP Referral to Treatment by a Specialist

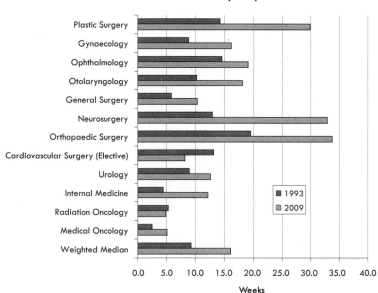

Source: Esmail, Nadeem, *Waiting Your Turn: Hospital Waiting Lists in Canada* (Vancouver: Fraser Institute, 2009 Report).

Canadians in need of medical care. Canadians can expect to wait long periods of time for diagnostic scans: in 2009, for example, the median national wait time for an MRI scan was 8.9 weeks, for a CT scan was 4.6 weeks, and for an ultrasound scan was 4.7 weeks.[14] Canadians also endure long waits for an appointment with a doctor when they are sick or needing care and to receive care in the emergency room, waits that are often much longer than those experienced by citizens of other nations that maintain universal approaches to health care insurance.[15] Critically, these wait times cause real harm to Canadians. Delays in diagnosis and treatment can be devastating for individuals, their families, their employers, and others who rely on them. Diseases might advance during the delay, thus potentially affecting the treatment and outcomes, while complications can also arise as a result of this deterioration.[16] Delays also lead to additional and often significant personal costs. Any wait time, even a short one, entails some amount of pain and suffering, mental anguish, lost productivity at work and leisure, and strained personal relationships. Wait times also take a toll on the family and friends of those waiting, and may even affect an individual's ability to provide for him or herself and loved ones.[17]

In part, Canada's long wait times for medical care result from a lack of medical resources. And this lack of medical resources is the result of Canada's governments having restricted the supply of medical professionals and purchases of medical technologies.

With regard to age-adjusted access to high-tech medical instruments, Canada performs dismally by comparison with other developed nations that maintain universal access health insurance systems. For example, while ranking number two as a health care spender in the most recent year for which comparable data are available, Canada ranked fourteenth of twenty-five in access to MRI machines (see Figure 8.3), nineteenth of twenty-six in access to CT scanners (see Figure 8.4), eighth of twenty-one in access to mammographys, and tied with New Zealand at nineteenth of twenty-one in access to lithotripters (see Figure 8.5).[18] For Canadians, this lack of medical technology not only means longer delays for diagnosis and treatment but also means that many Canadians receive a less sophisticated diagnosis than might be available otherwise because they are unable to secure an MRI or CT scan. In addition, many Canadians unnecessarily endure more invasive treatments because they cannot easily access technologies like lithotripters or PET scanners.

The problems caused by a lack of medical technology are compounded by the advanced age of much of Canada's technology inventory. For example, at the start of 2007, 30 percent of Canada's hospital-based MRI scanners, 46 percent of Canada's angiography suites, 42 percent of Canada's cardiac catheterization labs, and 42 percent of Canada's lithotripters were past their recommended lifecycles according to guidelines published by the Canadian Association of Radiologists.[19] Put simply, the limited inventory of technology that is in place in Canada is all too often old, outdated, and unsophisticated.

Canada's physician supply has also been limited by government's seeking to control health care expenditures. At the time of Medicare's inception, Canada maintained one

FIGURE 8.3
MRI machines per million population (age-adjusted) in select OECD countries, 2005

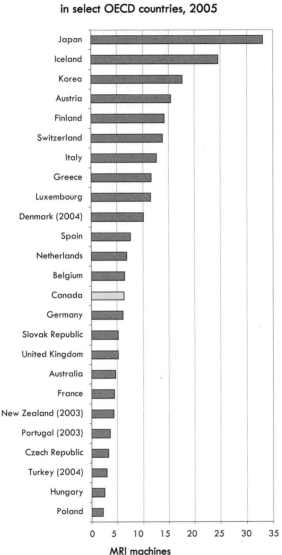

MRI machines

Source: Nadeem Esmail and Michael Walker, "How Good Is Canadian Health Care?" (Vancouver: Fraser Institute, 2008 Report).
Note: Figure for Turkey was not age-adjusted due to a low 65+ population not conducive to meaningful adjustment.

FIGURE 8.4
CT scanners per million population (age-adjusted) in select OECD countries, 2005

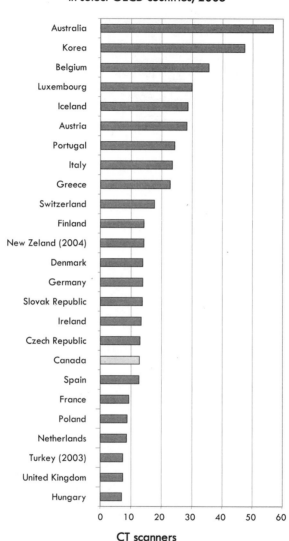

CT scanners

Source: Nadeem Esmail and Michael Walker, "How Good is Canadian Health Care?" (Vancouver: Fraser Institute, 2008 Report).

Notes: Japan is not included, as it has many more CT scanners (76.4 per million population in 2002) than other countries. Figure for Turkey was not age-adjusted due to a low 65+ population not conducive to meaningful adjustment.

FIGURE 8.5
Lithotripters per million population (age-adjusted) in select OECD countries, 2005

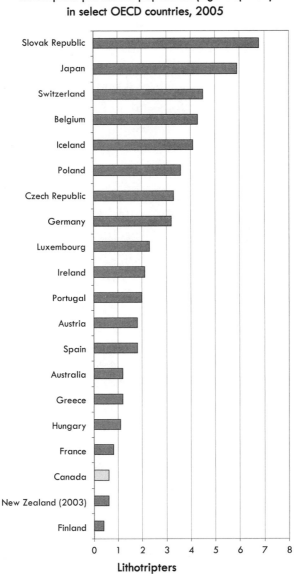

Lithotripters

Source: Nadeem Esmail and Michael Walker, "How Good Is Canadian Health Care?"
(Vancouver: Fraser Institute, 2008 Report).
Note: Korea is not included, as it has many more lithotripters
(13.5 per million population) than other countries

of the developed world's highest physician to population ratios on an age-adjusted basis.[20] Soon after however, some government officials and researchers voiced concern about the increasing number of physicians in Canada and its potential cost implications. These concerns eventually turned into reductions in medical school enrollment and post-graduate training positions and an intention to reduce Canada's reliance on foreign trained physicians over time.

Critically for Canadians, this policy regime has resulted in a physician-to-population ratio that ranks twenty-sixth among the twenty-eight developed nations that guarantee their citizens access to health care insurance regardless of ability to pay.[21] (See Table 8.1.) The consequences for those seeking care are increasingly clear in terms of both long wait times for access to physicians and in terms of the unavailability of regular family doctors. For example, in 2007 nearly 1.7 million Canadians aged twelve or older reported being unable to find a regular physician.[22] Similarly, a research poll completed in 2007 found that 14 percent of Canadians (approximately five million) were without a family doctor, more than 41 percent of whom (approximately two million) were unsuccessful in trying to find a family doctor.[23] And projections show that Canada's physician shortage will become much more acute in the coming years unless Canada becomes more reliant on foreign-trained physicians.[24]

Of course, there are those who will argue that many of these costs are acceptable because Canada's health care insurance system caters to all comers equally. This is also a misrepresentation of reality. A profusion of research reveals that cardiovascular surgery queues are routinely jumped by

TABLE 8.1: Physicians per 1,000 population (age-adjusted) in select OECD countries, 2006

Rank of 28	Country	
1	Iceland	4.5
2	Greece (2005)	4.4
3	Netherlands	4.0
4	Czech Republic	3.8
4	Norway	3.8
6	Belgium	3.7
6	Ireland	3.7
6	Slovak Republic (2004)	3.7
6	Switzerland	3.7
10	Denmark (2004)	3.6
11	Austria	3.4
11	Spain	3.4
13	France	3.2
13	Sweden (2005)	3.2
15	Australia (2005)	3.1
15	Italy	3.1
15	Germany	3.1
18	Portugal (2005)	3.0
19	Hungary	2.9
19	Luxembourg	2.9
21	New Zealand	2.7
22	Finland	2.6
23	Korea	2.4
23	Poland	2.4
23	United Kingdom	2.4
26	**Canada**	**2.3**
27	Japan	1.7
28	Turkey	1.6

Source: Esmail, Nadeem (2008). Canada's physician supply. *Fraser Forum* (November): 13–17.
Note: Figure for Turkey was not age-adjusted due to a low 65+ population not conducive to meaningful adjustment.

the famous and politically connected, that suburban and rural residents confront barriers to access not encountered by their urban counterparts, and that low-income Canadians have less access to specialists, particularly cardiovascular ones, are less likely to utilize diagnostic imaging, and have lower cardiovascular and cancer survival rates than their higher-income neighbors.[25] The truth is that the promise of equality in the Canadian system is not being realized in practice and that rationing by waiting in Canada is often a façade for a system of personal privilege.

This grim portrait is the legacy of a medical system offering low expectations cloaked in lofty rhetoric. The truth is that Canada's health care system is less a guiding light for reform and more an example of how not to structure a health care insurance system. More specifically, Canada's health care system and the trials and tribulations Canadians in need of medical care endure provide a clear lesson on the dire consequences of putting government in charge of health care.

NOTES

1. This term is not clearly defined in Canada, but instead is defined by each provincial government for its own tax-funded government health insurance program.

2. Although Canadian hospitals are legally considered private, not-for-profit entities, they are governed largely by a political process, given wage schedules for staff, are told when investment can be undertaken, denied the ability to borrow privately for investment, told which investments will be funded for operation, and forcibly merged or closed by provincial governments. They are considered, therefore, public hospitals for the sake of international comparability. Indeed, Detsky and

Naylor, in a discussion about the ownership status and structure of Canadian hospitals, state: "For all intents and purposes, they are public institutions," Detsky, Allan S. and C. David Naylor (2003). Canada's Health Care System—Reform Delayed. *NEJM* 349, 8: 804–10.

3. Nadeem Esmail and Michael Walker, "How Good is Canadian Health Care?" *Fraser Forum* (August 2002).

4. Brett J. Skinner, *Long-term or Short-term, Public Health Insurance is Not Sustainable: A Reply to CUPE About Health Spending Trends in Canada* (Vancouver: Fraser Institute, 2007).

5. Brett J. Skinner and Mark Rovere. *Paying More, Getting Less: Measuring the Sustainability of Government Health Spending in Canada* (Vancouver: Fraser Institute, 2009 Report).

6. Milagros Palacios, Niels Veldhuis, and Kumi Harischandra *Canadian Government Debt 2008: A Guide to the Indebtedness of Canada and the Provinces,* (Vancouver: Fraser Institute, 2008).

7. Canadian Institute for Health Information, *National Health Expenditure Trends, 1975–2009.* CIHI (2009).

8. Palacios et al, 2008.

9. Nadeem Esmail, *Waiting Your Turn: Hospital Waiting Lists in Canada* (Vancouver: Fraser Institute, 2009 Report).

10. Ibid.

11. Ibid.

12. See for example, Bacchus Barua and Nadeem Esmail, "Spend More, Wait Less?" *Fraser Forum* (February 2010): 16–26. It is worth noting that the Canadian Institute of Health Information found (not including the province of Quebec) that in 2007–2008, "Age-standardized rates of surgery outside the priority areas [hip and knee replacements, cataract surgery, cardiac revascularization, and cancer surgery] are about the same as they were in 2004–2005." (CIHI, *Surgical Volume Trends,* 2009:12.) Within the priority areas, rates of surgery climbed by 7 percent between 2004–2005 and 2005–2006, and then essentially stopped growing to 2007–2008. (CIHI, *Surgical Volume Trends*). Importantly, these non-increases occurred at the same time as provincial health spending per Canadian grew by about 9 percent (after accounting for inflation) between 2004 and 2007 (CIHI, *National Health Expenditure Trends*; calculations by author).

13. Esmail, *Waiting Your Turn.*

14. Ibid.

15. Cathy Schoen, Robin Osborn, Michelle M. Doty, Meghan Bishop, Jordon Peugh, and Nandita Murukutla, "Toward Higher-Performance Health Systems: Adults' Health Care Experiences in Seven Countries," *Health Affairs*, (2007): w717. (Web Exclusive), www.healthaffairs.org

16. Notably, Canada's medical specialists report clinically reasonable wait times that are much shorter than the actual wait times Canadians endure for scheduled or elective medical treatment. In 2009 for example, the median clinically reasonable wait for treatment after seeing a specialist across 12 major medical specialties was 5.8 weeks compared to an actual wait time from specialist to treatment of 8.0 weeks (Esmail, *Waiting Your Turn*).

17. For more on this see Esmail, *Waiting Your Turn* and Nadeem Esmail, "The Private Cost of Public Queues," *Fraser Forum* (November 2009): 32–36; and "The Economic Cost of Wait Times in Canada," Centre for Spatial Economics, 2008.

18. Esmail and Walker, 2008; In a non-age-adjusted comparison, Canada also ranked ninth of thirteen in access to PET scanners. Nadeem Esmail and Dominika Wrona, *Medical Technology in Canada*, (Vancouver: Fraser Institute, 2008).

19. Nadeem Esmail, *How Good is Canada's Medical Technology Inventory?* (Vancouver: Fraser Institute, 2008).

20. Esmail and Walker, 2008.

21. Nadeem Esmail, "Canada's Physician Supply," *Fraser Forum* (November 2009): 32–36.

22. Statistics Canada, Canadian Community Health Survey, *The Daily*, June 18, 2008.

23. College of Family Physicians of Canada (CFPC), "The College of Family Physicians of Canada Takes Action to Improve Access to Care for Patients in Canada," News release, October 11, 2007. www.cfpc.ca.

24. Esmail, "Canada's Physician Supply."

25. See for example David A. Alter, Antoni S. H. Basinski, and C. David Naylor, "A Survey of Provider Experiences and Perceptions of Preferential Access to Cardiovascular Care in Ontario, Canada," *Annals of Internal Medicine* 129 (1998): 567–72; Cynthia Ramsay, "Outside the City Walls: Not So Equal Access to Health Care in Canada. *Fraser Forum*

(January 1997): 19–23; Sheryl Dunlop, Peter C. Coyte, and Warren McIsaac, "Socio-economic Status and the Utilisation of Physicians' Services: Results from the Canadian National Population Health Survey," *Social Science and Medicine* (2000): 1–11; John J. You, Vikram Venkatesh, and Andreas Laupacis, "Better access to Outpatient Magnetic Resonance Imagining in Ontario—But for Whom?" *Open Medicine* 3 no. 1 (2009): 22–25; Sandor Demeter, Martin Reed, Lisa Lix, Leonard McWilliam, and William D. Leslie, "Socioeconomic Status and the Utilization of Diagnostic Imaging in an Urban Setting," *Canadian Medical Association Journal* 173, no. 10 (2005): 1173–7; David A. Alter, David Naylor, Peter Austin, and Jack V. Tu, "Effects of Socioeconomic Status on Access to Invasive Cardiac Procedures and on Mortality after Acute Myocardial Infarction," *New England Journal of Medicine* 341 (1999): 1359; and W. J. Mackillop, J. Zhang-Salomons; P. A. Groome; L. Paszat, and E. Holowaty, "Socioeconomic Status and Cancer Survival in Ontario," *Journal of Clinical Oncology* 15 (1997): 1680–9.

9

GOVERNMENT OVERSIGHT OF COMPARATIVE EFFECTIVENESS: LESSONS FROM WESTERN EUROPE

Helen Evans

P RESIDENT OBAMA has repeatedly emphasized the importance of limiting medical services to "health care that works." Although the president and his congressional supporters deny it, the fact is that government controlled rationing of health care is central to the Obama health plan. In June of 2009, the White House Council of Economic Advisers detailed the administration's goal of reducing health spending by 30 percent over the next two decades. Comparative effectiveness would be the vehicle used to eliminate "high cost, low-value treatments," with "performance measures" required by all health care providers. To identify such "high cost, low-value" care a

Helen Evans, PhD, is a citizen of the United Kingdom. A registered general nurse, she is the director of Nurses for Reform, a health fellow with the Adam Smith Institute, a senior fellow with the Libertarian Alliance, and a senior fellow with Progressive Vision—all with headquarters in London, England.

federal Coordinating Council for Comparative Effectiveness Research was funded in the $850 billion American Recovery and Reinvestment Act, the so-called economic stimulus bill, passed by the U.S. House of Representatives. The bill provided $1.1 billion for the new council, and delegated spending authority to the secretary of the Department of Health and Human Services (HHS) to investigate the effectiveness of different treatments by drugs and medical devices.

President Barack Obama's administration and Congress view comparative effectiveness as a key component of their highly interventionist health care plans because it gives government the ultimate authority to make official determinations of the clinical effectiveness and cost-effectiveness of medical treatments, procedures, drugs, and medical devices. Such statism will ultimately facilitate binding decisions on health plans and providers financed by federal taxpayers and, in time, potentially on private health insurance coverage too.

Of course, there is no reason why private-sector or government officials should not have access to the best information on what works and what doesn't. Nor is there any reason that such scientific evaluations should not be widely available to doctors, patients and other interested parties alike. But it is the contention of this author that studies of the comparative effectiveness of medical devices, drugs, and technology must be conducted primarily within the private sector and by medical experts rather than by government bodies, and that there should be no government influence over either the research or the distribution of information.

The key issue here is the personal liberty of patients to be able to choose the health care that, in the professional judgment of their doctors and advocates, best serves their own personal interests and not any broader, politically motivated agendas in the electoral spheres of politics. In this most personal part of life—the pursuit of health—it is essential that free individuals remain unburdened by the dictates and constraints of statist agendas.

MEDICAL TECHNOLOGY

Medical technology can be expensive. Over the past twenty years, health technology assessment (HTA)—the synthetic coordination of information assessing medicines and treatments—has become increasingly popular with policymakers and legislators around the world. Advocates of HTA invariably believe that such an approach has the capacity to provide decision-makers in the public and private sectors with objective information on the value of medical technologies, devices, and medicines. Driven by concerned perceptions of "unproven technology," "spiralling costs," and "increasing consumer expectations," its proponents aim to produce synthesised research information that they believe sheds light on the effects and costs of various forms of health technology.

Such an approach, however, guarantees the incremental advance of government control of private medical decisions and in so doing constrains private action. While formally said to be an instrument of efficiency and effectiveness, such approaches distort scientific research in the name of political or budgetary objectives while denying individual freedom of choice if those conducting the assessment are agencies intending to lower cost. It is in this sense that this approach places great power in the hands of government appointees and serves as a propaganda tool designed to legitimize anti-consumerist rationing.

AN INTRODUCTORY HISTORY OF COMPARATIVE EFFECTIVENESS IN HEALTH CARE

The intellectual roots of "effectiveness research" can be traced back to mid-18th century Scotland and the "arithmetical medicine" practiced by the graduates of the University of Edinburgh Medical School. It was there that James Lind famously undertook a controlled trial of six separate treatments for scurvy.[1] During the 1830s, Pierre Louis developed the méthode numérique in Paris, whereby he demonstrated that phlebotomy did not actually improve the survival rates of patients suffering from pneumonia.

At the beginning of the 20th century, Ernest Codman, an American physician, founded what is today known as "outcomes management" in patient care. This school was shunned by established institutions of the day, so Codman set up his own unit, the End Result Hospital. In line with his teachings and the findings from this unit, "end results" were made public in a privately published book, *A Study in Hospital Efficiency.*[2] Of 337 patients discharged from the hospital between 1911 and 1916, Codman recorded and publicized 123 medical errors.

In England, the 1930s saw the development of "health services research." In a world increasingly obsessed with egalitarian uniformity, J. A. Glover found a tenfold variation in the frequency of tonsillectomy.[3] Subsequently, following several decades of socialized health care in the United Kingdom, the 1970s and 1980s witnessed the release of a range of studies that highlighted wide geographical variations in general medical admissions including for operations such as appendectomy, caesarean section, cholecystectomy, hysterectomy, tonsillectomy, and prostatectomy.[4] Such variations not only demonstrated the inequities of the National Health Service (NHS), but also raised questions about the probity and cost-effectiveness of many of its treatments.

Following the publication of Archie Cochrane's *Effectiveness and Efficiency: Random Reflections on Health Services*[5] in the United States, researchers demonstrated large variations in the rates of prostatectomy for patients with benign prostatic hyperplasia.[6] This work and others suggested that such variations "meant either under-provision in some places and/or over-provision (and possibly ineffective treatment) in others."[7] While "comparative effectiveness" builds on skepticism, the investigation of variations, randomized control trials, and cost-benefit analysis, its reviews purport to be systematic. As such, they attempt to go beyond the more narrative-based reviews that used to dominate the typical review article in medical literature.

THE THINKING BEHIND
COMPARATIVE EFFECTIVENESS

In recent decades, health care has advanced in numerous ways. Across the developed world not only has medical knowledge progressed but investment in equipment and drugs has delivered unprecedented gains. Treatments are safer and more effective than ever before. Quality of life and life expectancy have been enhanced. Alongside aging populations has come the world of ever-increasing consumer expectations.

The rapid growth of medical knowledge and technology means it is much harder for physicians and health care providers to keep up-to-date. Indeed, the problem of information and practice transference is rendered almost impossible by the fact that health care is now also an increasingly statist and corporatist venture. Today, there is no such thing as a free market in health care, and many of the problems popularly associated with it are in fact the result of state failure.

Today, in virtually every country in the world, health care is heavily influenced by government, which oversees its professional monopolies through strict top-down regulation and control.[8] While there is nothing inherent in health care that demands such an approach, governments and politicians invariably make value judgments and grant legislative favor to interest groups, including doctors, nurses, and insurers, to whom they are beholden.

The idea that government is intrinsically a superior agent over and above a spontaneous and free market is groundless and misguided, particularly when one considers the extraordinarily personal decisions routinely required in health care. As David Friedman, a professor of law at Santa Clara University in California, has argued, both the notion of market failure in health economics and its popularity with most opinion leaders have arisen because many health policy analysts "interpret the problem in terms of fairness rather than efficiency."[9] This almost unconscious adherence to the notion of market failure in health care is rooted in:

> the error of judging a system by the comparison between its outcome and the best outcome that can be described, rather than judging it by a comparison between its outcome and the outcome that would actually be produced by the best alternative system available. If, as seems likely, all possible sets of institutions fall short of producing perfect outcomes, then a policy of comparing observed outcomes to ideal ones will reject any existing system . . . The question we should ask, and try to answer, is not what outcome would be ideal but what outcome we can expect from each of various alternative sets of institutions, and which, from that limited set of alternatives, we prefer . . . My conclusion is that there is no good reason to expect government involvement in the medical market, either the extensive involvement that now exists or the still more extensive involvement that many advocated, to produce desirable results.[10]

Curiously, it is within the context of government control and anti-competitive corporatism that new and innovative medical treatments are met with initiatives for even more rationing by government officials, as well as other highly regulated players including private medical insurers.

In recent years, many countries have introduced comparative effectiveness or HTA programs. In reality, many politicians and officials have done so not least because they are trying to get themselves off the hook for past promises their forebears made concerning the provision of comprehensive, unlimited, or, as in the case of the United Kingdom, seemingly "free" health care at the point of service.

Because extensive government intervention has destroyed genuine health care markets and has made it impossible for individuals to determine a clear and transparent value of the costs and benefits of health care technology through a normally functioning price system, the proponents of comparative effectiveness, or health technology assessment, have instead resorted to a predictably pseudoscientific methodology to give their bureaucratic determinations a sheen of objectivity. As with other forms of centralized government planning, the practitioners of these bureaucratic dark arts attempt to capture and mathematically model their assessments. In assessing health technology, they seek "to compare and prioritize new technologies based on different units that aggregate . . . benefits."[11]

In a study of HTA for the Stockholm Network, a European think tank, research has focused on these assessments in terms of the value of human life:

> In HTA, the dominant aggregate natural unit is called
> quality-adjusted life years (QALYs). Generally, QALYs
> factor in both the quantity and the quality of life generated
> by new health care interventions. It is the arithmetic calcu-
> lation of life expectancy and a measure of the quality of the

remaining life years . . . To date QALYs are the preferred
indicator of HTA calculations, although one may find additional tools in use by HTA bodies such as HRQOL ('health
related quality of life,' which considers physical function,
social function, cognitive function, distress, pain—in brief,
anything to do with quality of life), DALYs ('disability
adjusted life years'—life lost due to premature mortality in
the population and the years lost due to disability for inci-
dents of the studied health condition), and healthy-year
equivalents (HYEs).[12]

Despite the pretense of scientific objectivity, this type of
health technology assessment is nothing of the sort. It is
designed primarily to provide policymakers with a legiti-
mizing rubric by which they can mimic a few elements of
the market and therefore deploy a degree of fake economic
rationality in justifying their decisions. In this way, practitioners of HTA attempt to balance the requirement to
provide innovative health care technologies with inherently uninformed efforts at controlling the costs of those
technologies.

Consider the quality of human life and lifespan. The use
of QALYs is pseudoscience. It is nothing more than a tool
for central planning that attempts to objectify what is inherently subjective. The limited attempts to capture accurately
the various "units of health care benefit" mean that there is
an inevitable gulf between the theoretical underpinnings of
QALYs and the actual behavior of ordinary people.

Moreover, the artificial prioritization of so-called cost-
based considerations by practitioners of health technology

assessment is invariably made at the expense of other considerations. As Dr. Meir Pugatch and Francesca Ficai of the Stockholm Network note, "Thus, a decision to prioritize a less therapeutically effective medicine because of cost-based considerations over an effective, but more expensive, medicine could lead to some serious political, social and moral dilemmas."[13]

Not only is this type of health technology assessment methodologically flawed but it is incompatible with personal freedom and contradicts the subjective choices of genuine economic agents. When deployed at the national level through the power of a government agency, it is inevitably subject to additional political pressures. Indeed, in 2010, it is clear that national organizations that conduct these assessments—such as the National Institute for Health and Clinical Excellence in the United Kingdom or the Institute for Quality and Efficiency in Health Care in Germany—are in the business of rationing health care technologies so that they mesh with the politically fixed budgetary allocations of the national government.

HOW COMPARATIVE EFFECTIVENESS REALLY WORKS IN WESTERN EUROPE

According to the International Network of Agencies for Health Technology Assessments (INAHTA),[14] many industrialized countries have bodies that are charged with health technology assessments or comparative effectiveness studies. Despite this, the evolution of these bodies and their responsibilities at the national decision-making level has been far from uniform. For example, some of these bodies have an advisory role. They make reimbursements or pricing recommendations to a national or regional governing body, as is the case in Denmark. Others have a more explicit regulatory role. They are accountable to government ministers and are responsible for listing and pricing medicines and devices. This is the case in France, Germany, and the United Kingdom.

The United Kingdom

The experience of the United Kingdom in making the difficult decisions about what kind of health care technologies, devices, drugs, and medical treatments and procedures should be favored in Britain's National Health Service has been cited favorably by some in the United States.

Yet, the NHS was established in 1948. It is a single-payer health care system, directly administered by the British government, funded through taxation, and provided mainly by public-sector institutions. Because the NHS is a fully nationalized entity, the central government specifies the capital and current budgets of its regional health authorities and determines the expenditure on drugs by controlling the budgets given to each general practitioner. Overall, NHS health care is rationed through long waiting lists and, in some cases, omission of various treatments.[15]

For the British government, the practice of HTA facilitates rationing by delay. It is a tool that aims to ensure that expensive new technologies are initially provided only in hospitals that have the technical capacity to evaluate them. While the NHS Research and Development Health Technology Assessment Programme is funded by the Department of Health and, according to its criteria, researches the costs, effectiveness, and impact of health technologies, the Medicines and Healthcare Products Regulatory Agency (MHRA) ensures that drugs and devices are safe.[16]

In 1999, the government went a step further and set up the National Institute for Health and Clinical Excellence (NICE).[17] At its heart is the Centre for Health Technology Evaluation that issues formal guidance on the use of new and existing medicines based on rigid and proscriptive "economic" and clinical formulas. With the NHS obliged to adhere to NICE's pronouncements, criticism of NICE has been ceaseless, particularly from various patient organizations.

NICE is a controversial body. It has tried repeatedly to stop breast cancer patients from receiving the powerful breakthrough drug Herceptin and patients with Alzheimer's disease from receiving the drug Aricept. The criteria by which this agency makes its decisions have been kept largely secret from the public. As is inevitable with any nationalized health care system, life-extending medicines such as those to treat renal cancers are refused on the grounds of limited resources and the need to make decisions based not on genuine market economics but on an artificial assessment of the benefit that may be gained by the patient and society "as a whole."

In 2001, NICE deliberately restricted state-insured sufferers of multiple sclerosis from receiving the innovative medicine beta interferon. Claiming that its relatively high price jeopardized the efficacy of the NHS, NICE told patients with the more severe forms of the disease that they would have to go on suffering in the name of politically defined equity.[18]

In more recent years, patients with painful and debilitating forms of rheumatoid arthritis have been informed in many instances by NICE that they will not be allowed to receive a sequential range of medicines that often have been proved to be of significant benefit. Instead, the institute decreed that "people will be prevented from trying a second anti-TNF arthritis treatment if the first does not work for their condition."[19]

Similarly, in August 2008, patients with kidney cancer continued to be denied effective treatments designed to prolong their lives, often by months or even a few years. The calculations used by NICE have been systematically disputed by clinical experts who are more concerned with patient welfare than with political vote-seeking, but the institute has also come under fire for not involving doctors who are active on the front line of medicine: "With Sutent [a kidney cancer treatment] for instance, there was just one oncologist on the panel."[20]

In January 2009, patients with osteoporosis also fell afoul of NICE. The institute declared that only a small minority of patients with this debilitating disease would receive the medicine Protelos, and even they would receive it only as an extreme last resort. While clinicians and osteoporosis support groups have pointed out that more than 70,000 hip fractures result in 13,000 premature deaths in the UK each year and that these otherwise avoidable episodes needlessly cost the NHS billions of pounds, not only are patients being denied necessary treatments, but taxpayers' money is wasted.[21]

Indeed, according to its annual reports and accounts, NICE is now spending more money on communicating its decisions than would be spent if it allowed patients access to many of the medicines it is so busy denying them. The money that the institute now spends on public relations campaigns "could have paid for 5,000 Alzheimer's sufferers to get £2.50-a-day drugs for a year," according to the *Daily Mail.*[22]

Devoid of a genuine free market and its price signals, this top-down system ironically ignores many of the societal costs, such as illness-related unemployment, associated with failure to treat severe illness. Moreover, the fact that preventing access to more costly medicines may save money in the short term overlooks the costs for the future. If older medicines lead to more rapid deterioration of a condition, the effect could be a more expensive hospital or nursing home episode later.

Denmark

The Danish health care system is completely state-funded, with public provision of hospital beds representing more than 90 percent of the hospital sector. Under the Healthcare Act, citizens are covered for all or part of expenditures for treatment, including reimbursement for all pharmaceutical products listed with the Danish Medicines Agency. Therefore, there is no need for price regulation of drugs. With central and municipal government having significant control of the funding and provision of health care, the acquisition of new technology is left initially to the five regions' administrations that run the hospitals.

Denmark's national HTA system was explicitly established on the basis of its making prioritized resource-allocation decisions. These decisions are carried out by the unit known as the Danish Centre for Evaluation and Health Technology Assessment (DACEHTA), which operates within the framework of the National Board of Health (NBH), itself a part of the Danish Ministry of Health.[23] In reality, this means that "[t]he Ministry keeps a close watch on it in order to neutralize 'expensive' healthcare technologies, as their adoption results in requests for extra funding from the regions."[24]

France

In France, health care is a statutory right enshrined in the Constitution of the Fifth Republic. Unlike in Denmark or the United Kingdom however, French health care is financed mainly by social insurance and delivered by a mixture of public and private providers. While two-thirds of French hospitals are state-owned, one-third are private, with half of the latter group being not-for-profit.

There have been various attempts in recent years to extend government control of health care costs. In 1991, the French government extended the Health Map system by which it controls the capital construction of all hospitals as well as their budgets, the purchase of medical equipment, the rates charged by private hospitals, the number of pharmacies per head, and even the price of drugs.[25]

In 2005, the government went a stage further with the establishment of a centralized High Health Authority. While this body has had only a limited impact—and France continues to enjoy a comparatively higher diffusion rate for new technologies than is found in many other countries in Europe—it is nevertheless designed to stipulate the benefits of medicines and determine their price-reimbursement levels. As such, it is set to raise the focus on cost-containment and to bring its decision-making under closer state control.

Germany

As in France, health care in Germany is financed primarily by social insurance and provided by a mixture of public and private providers. While all services are contracted instead of being provided directly by the government, more than 10 percent of Germans opt for full private medical insurance.[26] Providing a potent incentive for people to exit state health care, the regulated private sector puts pressure on the government to ensure that the sectorial differences in service do not become so wide that ever-larger numbers of young, high-income consumers defect by going private and delegitimizing a central pillar of the Bismarckian welfare state.

While the pressure to maintain some semblance of parity with the private sector meant that state spending rose dramatically for many years after the introduction of a formal reference pricing system in 1989, the strategic objective of the German Ministry of Health has been to reduce supply,

particularly through the use of published positive and negative lists concerning medicines and treatments. Through
these lists, pressure is applied to the statutory sick funds to
control costs.[27]

It is in this context that health technology assessment
has played an ever-greater role in German health policy
since the 1990s. In 1990, the Office of Technology Assessment at the German Parliament (TAB) was established, and
in 2004, the government set up the Institute for Quality and
Economic Efficiency in the Healthcare Sector (IQWiG).

Tasked with the central goal of efficiency, IQWiG investi-
gates and stipulates which therapeutic and diagnostic services are appropriate.[28] It disseminates its pronouncements
to a variety of so called "self-governing bodies," which use
such information in their benefits catalogs. Being funded
primarily by the German Ministry for Health and Social
Affairs, assessment bodies can refuse a hospital's claim for
reimbursement for the unauthorized use of new technology.

LESSONS FOR AMERICA

There is a pervasive European mythology that American
health care is rooted in the free market, and moreover that
any and all problems in the American health system can be
traced to its free market approach. In reality of course,
much of American health care has long been a highly
planned, regulated, and government-funded system. Today,
the trajectory towards ever-greater health statism has never
looked so strong. Through major entitlement and welfare

programs such as Medicare and Medicaid, which contribute to rapidly growing American health care costs, the health care system takes a historically higher proportion of gross domestic product than does even the British NHS. Moreover, by virtue of the structure and financing of private-sector health insurance, there is little consumer control over health care dollars.

Nonetheless, the United States is not only a major consumer of health care services, but it is also the world's largest producer of medical technology. Investment in new medical technology is comparatively high, as is its rate of diffusion: "This is demonstrated by cross-national examinations of the comparative availability of selected medical technologies such as radiation therapy and open-heart surgery. Measured in units per million, the United States experiences levels of availability up to three times greater than in Canada and Germany."[29]

Fearing the impact of the rising costs of Medicare, Medicaid, and the highly regulated arrangements of the private insurance sector, top policymakers in Washington, DC are clearly committed to the idea of institutional arrangements that would make top-down pronouncements on the cost-effectiveness of new medical technologies. The idea of statutorily created agencies charged with system-wide cost containment and rationing of medical services and technologies is becoming surprisingly fashionable in the world's elite policy circles.

The implications of this trend are alarming for U.S. citizens, particularly when one considers that the technology a society uses reflects the wider and underlying incentive structures it adopts for using it: "An incentive structure that encourages providers to trade off the costs and benefits of health care gives providers little incentive to use expensive technologies and thus researchers will have little incentive to create it."[30]

In the long term, a statist, centralized control of medical technology offers little if any regulatory benefit. Through its own logic, it not only stifles innovation, but it also ends up precluding those very inventions that could turn out to be of immeasurable benefit to individuals and to society in general. If comparative effectiveness and health technology assessment are to be useful, they must be generated primarily by independent academics and the private sector on a competitive and non-coercive basis.

In thinking about comparative effectiveness, America should learn key lessons from failures in Western Europe and it should be guided by three principles:

1. America should reject the statutory creation of any organization that seeks to centralize government control of patient access to drugs, devices, medical technologies, treatments, or procedures.
2. Comparative effectiveness research in health care and health technology assessments should be undertaken only by the private sector and not governmental bodies.
3. Comparative effectiveness research should be patient-centered and supportive of quality and value, not focused simply on cost-containment. In this respect, it should promote scientific advances, health information technology, and the emerging science of personalized medicine.

CONCLUSION

As is clear from the British experience and other examples in Western Europe, a comparative effectiveness strategy that relies on central planning and coercion will not only be counterproductive in the long run—because it will undermine the incentives for medical innovation—but it will also lead to the imposition of cost constraints that will worsen patients' medical conditions and damage the quality of their lives.

NOTES

1. Stephen R. Brown, *Scurvy: How a Surgeon, a Mariner, and a Gentleman Solved the Greatest Medical Mystery of the Age of Sail* (New York: St. Martin's Press, 2003).

2. Ernest A. Codman, *A Study in Hospital Efficiency* (Boston, Mass.: Privately printed, 1916).

3. J. A. Glover, "The Incidence of Tonsillectomy in School Children," *Proceedings of the Royal Society of Medicine*, XXXI (1938): 1219–1236.

4. D. Sanders, A. Coulter, K. McPherson, *Variations in Hospital Admission Rates: A Review of the Literature* (London: King Edward's Hospital Fund for London, 1989), 31.

5. Archie Cochrane, *Effectiveness and Efficiency: Random Reflections on Health Services* (Leeds: Nuffield Provincial Hospitals Trust, 1972).

6. J. E. Wennberg, A. G. Mulley, D. Hanley, et al., "An Assessment of Prostatectomy for Benign Urinary Tract Obstruction: Geographic Variations and the Evaluation of Medical Care Outcomes," *JAMA*, 259, no. 20 (1988): 3027–3030.

7. Andrew Stevens, Ruairidh Milne, and Amanda Burls, "Health Technology Assessment: History and Demand," *Journal of Public Health Medicine*, 25, no. 2 (1998): 99.

8. Brian Micklethwait, "How and How Not to Demonopolise Medicine," *Political Notes* 56, Libertarian Alliance, London, 1991.

9. David Friedman, "Should Medicine Be a Commodity? An Economist's Perspective," *Philosophy and Medicine: Rights to Health Care* 38 (1991), at www.daviddfriedman.com/Academic/Medicine_Commodity/Medicine_Commodity.html (January 29, 2009).

10. Ibid.

11. Meir P. Pugatch and Francesca Ficai, "A Healthy Market? An Introduction to Health Technology Assessment," Stockholm Network, London (2007): 5.

12. Ibid.

13. Ibid. 6.

14. See INAHTA home page at www.inahta.org (January 30, 2009).

15. Helen Evans, *Sixty Years On—Who Cares for the NHS?* (London: Institute of Economic Affairs, 2008): 26–54.

16. See MHRA home page at www.mhra.gov.uk (January 30, 2009).

17. Pugatch and Ficai, "A Healthy Market? An Introduction to Health Technology Assessment," 8.

18. "MS Research Urges End of NHS Bar on Drug," *The Daily Telegraph*, June 19, 2001.

19. See press release, "NICE Limits Options for People with Rheumatoid Arthritis," Arthritis Cares, London, July 21, 2008.

20. "Nasty Truth About NICE: It's the Body that Rations NHS Drugs. But This Leading Cancer Specialist Says Its Decisions Are Deeply Flawed," *The Daily Mail*, August 8, 2008.

21. "NICE Decision to Block Osteoporosis Drug Access Was 'Irrational,'" *The Daily Telegraph*, January 20, 2009.

22. "Drug Watchdog NICE 'Spends More on "Spin" than Tests on New Treatments,'" *The Daily Mail*, September 10, 2008, at www.daily mail.co.uk/health/article-1054049/Drug-watchdog-NICE-spends-spin -tests-new-treatments.html (January 30, 2009).

23. See National Board of Health home page at www.sst.dk (January 30, 2009).

24. Meir P. Pugatch and Helen Davison, "A Healthy Market? Health Assessment Technology in Context," Stockholm Network, London, (2007): 9.

25. Brian Abel-Smith and Elias Mossialos, "Cost Containment and Health Care Reform: A Study of the European Union," London School of Economics and Political Science *Occasional Paper in Health Policy* 2, (1994): 33–35.

26. Pugatch and Davison, "A Healthy Market? Health Assessment Technology in Context," p. 10.

27. Ibid., 11.

28. Ibid.

29. "American Democracy and Health Care," *British Journal of Political Science* 27, no. 4 (October 1997): 573.

30. Pugatch and Davison, "A Healthy Market? Health Assessment Technology in Context," 16.

ABOUT THE
CONTRIBUTING AUTHORS

Scott W. Atlas is a senior fellow at the Hoover Institution, a professor at the Stanford University Medical Center, and a senior fellow at the Freeman Spogli Institute for International Studies. Atlas's research interests are domestic and global health care policy, particularly the role of government in pricing, quality, access, and innovation. During the 2008 campaign, Atlas was a senior adviser and coordinator of the Health Policy Team for one of the major presidential candidates. At Freeman Spogli, he studies health systems of emerging economies; he also participated in the World Bank's Commission on Growth and Development. He lectures throughout the world on MRI advances and key economic issues related to technology innovation. Atlas has received numerous awards and honors; he has also been a member of the Nominating Committee for the Nobel Prize in Medicine and Physiology for several years. Atlas received his BS from the University of Illinois Urbana-Champaign and his MD from the University of Chicago.

Richard A. Epstein has been the Peter and Kirsten Bedford Senior Fellow at the Hoover Institution since 2000. He is now the Laurence A. Tisch Professor of Law at New York University and the James Parker Hall Distinguished Service Professor of Law at the University of Chicago. He has been a member of the American Academy of Arts and Sciences since 1985 and a senior fellow of the Center for Clinical Medical Ethics at the University of Chicago School of Medicine from 1983 to the present. He served as editor of the *Journal of Legal Studies* from 1981 to 1991 and of the *Journal of Law and Economics* from 1991 to 2001. His books include *Overdose: How Excessive Government Regulation*

Stifles Pharmaceutical Innovation (Yale, 2006) and *Mortal Peril: Our Inalienable Rights to Health Care?* (Addison-Wesley, 1997).

Nadeem Esmail is a senior fellow at the Fraser Institute in Canada. He is the institute's former director of Health System Performance Studies, and former manager of the Alberta Policy Research Centre. He completed his BA (honors) in economics at the University of Calgary and received an MA in economics from the University of British Columbia. While on staff at the institute, Esmail authored or coauthored more than thirty comprehensive studies and more than 150 articles on a wide range of health care topics, including waiting lists, international comparisons of health care systems, hospital report cards, medical technology, and the physician shortage. His articles have appeared in newspapers across North America, including the *National Post, Globe and Mail, National Review Online,* and *Wall Street Journal.* He has also spoken internationally on health care policy and reform.

Helen Evans is a senior health policy expert and a registered nurse with a wealth of clinical and health care delivery experience. She is currently director of Nurses for Reform, a health fellow with the Adam Smith Institute, a senior fellow with both Progressive Vision and the Libertarian Alliance, and a director of the leading predictive public affairs consultancy, Farsight SPI Ltd. A former university guest lecturer, she has an extensive background in British and European health policy and a detailed knowledge of the history of the National Health Service. A graduate in health management, she was awarded a PhD in health economics from Brunel University in 2006. Having previously worked with Stockholm Network in London and for the Centre for the New Europe in Brussels, over the years her nursing career has seen her work as a senior nurse in some of Britain's most prestigious hospitals, including the Royal London Hospitals Trust and St. Bartholomew's. Today she lives in London with her husband, daughter, and three cats.

Scott Gottlieb is a practicing physician and resident fellow at the American Enterprise Institute. From 2005 to 2007, Dr. Gottlieb served as FDA deputy commissioner at the Food and Drug Administration (FDA) and, before that, as a senior adviser to the FDA commissioner and as the FDA's director of Medical Policy Development. He also worked on implementing the new Medicare drug benefit as a senior adviser to the administrator of Center of Medicare and Medicaid Services (CMS). Dr. Gottlieb continues to practice medicine as a hospitalist. He completed a residency in internal medicine at New York's Mount Sinai Hospital and is a graduate of the Mount Sinai School of Medicine and Wesleyan University, Middletown, Connecticut.

Douglas Holtz-Eakin is currently the president of the American Action Forum and a commissioner on the congressionally chartered Financial Crisis Inquiry Commission. He served as the director of domestic and economic policy for John McCain's 2008 presidential campaign. Holtz-Eakin was the sixth director of the nonpartisan Congressional Budget Office and served as the chief economist of the President's Council of Economic Advisers from 2001 to 2002. He was a senior fellow at the Peter G. Peterson Institute for International Economics (2007–08), the director of the Maurice R. Greenberg Center for Geoeconomic Studies, and the Paul A. Volcker Chair in International Economics at the Council on Foreign Relations.

Roger Stark is a retired cardiac surgeon who has dealt with Medicare, Medicaid, private insurance companies, HMOs, and the uninsured. He is currently employed as a health care analyst for the Washington Policy Center in Seattle. Dr. Stark has served on the Governing Board of Overlake Hospital in Bellevue, Washington, and is the past chairman of Overlake's Foundation Board. An active member of the Woodinville Rotary, he has also been a member of many professional organizations. He is the author of the book *Health Care in the US Today: Problems and Solutions.*

Grace-Marie Turner is president of the Galen Institute, a public policy research organization that she founded in 1995 to promote an informed debate over free-market ideas for health reform. She speaks and writes extensively about incentives to promote a more competitive, consumer-driven marketplace in the health sector. She also is founder and facilitator of the Health Policy Consensus Group, which serves as a forum for analysts from market-oriented think tanks around the country to analyze and develop health policy recommendations. She is the editor of *Empowering Health Care Consumers through Tax Reform*, which explains that tax reform can lead to a better-functioning market in the health sector, and she produces a widely read weekly electronic newsletter, *Health Policy Matters*. She received the 2007 Outstanding Achievement Award for Promotion of Consumer Driven Health Care from Consumer Health World.

Glen Whitman is a professor of economics at California State University, Northridge and an adjunct scholar with the Cato Institute. He received his PhD in economics from New York University in 2000. His research in applied game theory, economic analysis of law, and economic methodology has been published in the *Journal of Legal Studies*, *International Review of Law and Economics*, *UCLA Law Review*, and other scholarly journals. His current policy interests include health care and paternalistic legislation.

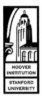

WORKING GROUP ON HEALTH CARE POLICY

The WORKING GROUP ON HEALTH CARE POLICY will aim to devise public policies that enable more Americans to get better value for their health care dollar and foster appropriate innovation that extends and improves life. Key principles that guide policy formation include the central role of individual choice and competitive markets in financing and delivering health services, individual responsibility for health behaviors and decisions, and appropriate guidelines for government intervention in health care markets.

The core membership of this working group includes Scott W. Atlas, John F. Cogan, R. Glenn Hubbard, Daniel P. Kessler, Mark V. Pauly, and Charles E. Phelps.

INDEX